A Medical Teacher's Manual for Success

A Medical Teacher's Manual for Success

 Five Simple Steps

Helen M. Shields, M.D., FACP, AGAF

Associate Professor of Medicine
Associate Master, Oliver Wendell Holmes Society
Harvard Medical School
Physician
Beth Israel Deaconess Medical Center
Boston, Massachusetts

The Johns Hopkins University Press
Baltimore

The Johns Hopkins University Press
2715 North Charles Street
Baltimore, Maryland 21218-4363
www.press.jhu.edu

Library of Congress Cataloging-in-Publication Data
Shields, Helen M.
   A medical teacher's manual for success : five simple steps /
Helen M. Shields.
       p. ; cm.
   Includes bibliographical references and index.
   ISBN-13: 978-0-8018-9766-5 (pbk. : alk. paper)
   ISBN-10: 0-8018-9766-1 (pbk. : alk. paper)
   1. Medicine—Study and teaching. 2. Medical colleges—
Faculty. 3. Medical teaching personnel. I. Title.
   [DNLM: 1. Education, Medical—methods. 2. Teaching—
methods. 3. Education, Medical—organization &
administration. 4. Faculty, Medical. W 18 S555m 2011]
   R737.S47 2011
   610.71'1—dc22   2010013977

A catalog record for this book is available from the
British Library.

*Special discounts are available for bulk purchases of this book. For
more information, please contact Special Sales at 410-516-6936 or
specialsales@press.jhu.edu.*

To my devoted husband and best friend, Richard A. Aparo, whose consistently wise advice has helped me to succeed

To my son Christopher Shields Aparo, an ideal pupil, whose eagerness to learn and excellent questions stimulated me to teach

To my wonderful parents, Walter A. Shields and Helen M. Shields, who gave me enormous encouragement and support

To my four sisters, Virginia Shields Walker, Eileen Shields West, Joan Shields, and Loraine Shields, each of whom has inspired me to be a more creative and caring teacher

Contents

Preface

I have written this book to help other teachers succeed in being better teachers; have more fun and less apprehension about teaching the art and science of medicine; achieve their goal of receiving accolades from their peers, fellows, residents, and students; win teaching awards or prizes; publish their teaching methods and educational projects; and, finally, be promoted.

I follow a framework of five simple steps for each teaching assignment, whether it be a lecture, a small group, or a workshop. These steps, which are discussed in detail in chapter 4, are the essential tools for teaching memorable learning sessions and ensuring success.

Acknowledgments

It is impossible to thank all the teachers, colleagues, and assistants who have helped and influenced me. I want to acknowledge, though, some of the institutions to which I owe my success, including Tufts University Medical School in Boston, University of Pennsylvania Medical School in Philadelphia, New York Hospital–Cornell Medical College in New York City, Mount Holyoke College in South Hadley, Massachusetts, Washington University Medical School in St. Louis, the Mary Louis Academy in Jamaica, New York, and Harvard Medical School and Beth Israel Deaconess Medical Center in Boston, Massachusetts. I also want to recognize the many people who helped me become successful.

My administrators have helped me balance my clinical responsibilities with my teaching career. From 1993 to 2002, Jeanne Crowgey enabled me to focus on directing and teaching the gastrointestinal pathophysiology course through her extraordinary ability to juggle my clinical practice and teaching duties, helping me behind the scenes at every turn. I am indebted to Jeanne for her vision, constant encouragement, excellent suggestions, high energy, marvelous manner of speaking with patients, and pragmatic advice. Susan Rakich Rizzo, MPH, my excellent administrator from 2002 to 2005, improved the teaching in the pathophysiology course and in my other teaching presentations with her outstanding computer skills and practical suggestions. From 2005 to 2009, Andrea Lenco, MPH, provided key support for my academic projects with her expert computer skills and wise advice. Francisca Xavier-Depina, my current administrator, deftly, capably, and expertly helps me balance, on a daily basis, my clinical, teaching, and research responsibilities through her tireless efforts, unusually strong work ethic, outstanding interpersonal skills, and extraordinary kindness and attention to my patients.

I am grateful to my good friends and consistent supporters, Natalie Wolf and the late Leo E. Wolf, whose confidence in me as a medical teacher led to their funding the gastrointestinal pathophysiology course tutorial schematics yearly since 2002 for each second-year student at Harvard Medical School.

My longtime friend and colleague, Ashok Sen Gupta, PhD, encouraged me to write and has provided advice about writing style; I am deeply in his debt, as I am to Miriam S. Wetzel, PhD, who taught me the basics of course organization, essential tips and specific directions for problem-based learning tutorials, small-group exercises, mini-cases, focused discussions, and multistation exercises. In addition, Dr. Wetzel showed me how to write problem-based learning cases, create learning objectives, seek memorable visual images, and organize faculty development meetings. I admire her genuinely kind, welcoming, and humble manner and have consciously tried to emulate her style.

Jane N. Hayward, of the Media Services Department at Beth Israel Deaconess Medical Center, has been a marvelous collaborator who has helped translate my vision for pathophysiologic "placemats" into a reality as well as improve each of my teaching presentations and educational research data.

I am deeply grateful to Donna Wolfe, MFA, for sharing her expertise on how to properly format and present a curriculum vitae for promotion on the teacher-clinician track.

I acknowledge the invaluable assistance, creative ideas, and intellectual energy of each of my outstanding teaching fellows. In chronological order, I thank Eric Goldberg, MD, Samuel Somers, MD, MMSc, Win Travassos, MD, Sonal Patel Ullman, MD, Seema Maroo, MD, Daniel Leffler, MD, MA, Richard Paul O'Farrell, MBBS, Paola Blanco, MD, Stephen Kappler, MD, Tyler Berzin, MD, MMS, and Sarah Flier, MD. I also thank my outstanding abdominal exam teaching fellow, Nielsen Fernandez-Becker, MD, PhD, and Melissa Tukey, MD, the abdominal exam resident for their outstanding help. I am indebted to Marika McGrath, MA, Intercultural Relations, for her organizational skills and terrific help with the "Healing Healthcare Disparities through Education" workshops.

Particular thanks go to Daniel Leffler, MD, MA, for encouraging me to write up my educational research projects and for helping me write better. I am grateful to Steven Kappler, MD, for his excellent advice about audience-response systems.

Since 2002, I, along with my teaching fellows, have been privileged to observe David Garvin, PhD, teach Harvard Business School classes, and have learned, from his superb case-based teaching. We have also watched other outstanding professors at Harvard Business School, including, in chronological order, Jay Lorsch, PhD, Jack Gabarro, PhD, Michael Tushman, PhD, and Thomas DeLong, PhD.

I am also indebted to Thomas DeLong, PhD, of Harvard Business School, for supporting me and my teaching projects, teaching me how to teach better, listening to my questions, providing wise and practical answers, and lending his terrific teaching talents to the integration of cross-cultural care across all four years of medical school.

Michele Cohn, Andrea Lenco, MPH, and Sheila Salamone, the wonderfully responsive and intelligent course managers at Harvard Medical School, have meticulously organized the gastrointestinal pathophysiology course.

I thank James Honan, EdD, of Harvard University's Graduate School of Education, for his valuable teaching on the art of questioning, and Brian Mandell, PhD, of Harvard University's John F. Kennedy School of Government, for his discussion of summarizing, and Janet Hafler, EdD, who helped me change the role of the tutor from that of a facilitator to that of a discussion leader and whose talents at managing group dynamics have been a terrific model to follow. I am also grateful to Samuel Somers, MD, MMSc, Barbara Nath, MD, and Laurie Raymond, MD, for creating and participating in annual faculty development exercises to help tutors become discussion leaders, and to Daniel Guss, MD, who, as a second-year tutorial student, was instrumental in our successfully changing the tutor to a discussion leader. Lee Warren, PhD, of the Derek Bok Center for Teaching and Learning at Harvard University, gave me valuable advice, practical and influential teaching videos, and books from the Derek Bok Center.

Daniel Federman, MD, is my role model for being an expert consultant on an inpatient service and for organizing and running an effective and efficient faculty meeting. I am grateful to Arvind Agnihotri, MD, Cecil Coggins, MD, Douglas Drachman, MD, and Farouc Jaffer, MD, PhD, for being outstanding role models for physician-patient communication skills at the bedside and in the office setting.

I deeply appreciate the opportunity that Dr. Federman gave me when he placed me on the newly formed Dean's Committee for Excellence in Tutoring.

I am grateful to Stephen Krane, MD, and Elaine Glebus for appointing me to the position of senior fellow of the Walter Bradford Cannon Society; this position gave me understanding of the society system at Harvard Medical School and the importance of advising students and was a stepping stone to my being named to the associate master position in the Oliver Wendell Holmes Society.

My thanks to Augustus White III, MD, PhD, for appointing me to the associate master position of the Oliver Wendell Holmes Society in 2001 and for asking me to integrate cross-cultural care into the gastrointestinal pathophysiology course in 2005. Dr. White has been my role model for a mentor. I am grateful to Anthony D'Amico, MD, PhD, for his consistent encouragement, support, and advice, first as an associate master and now as master of the Oliver Wendell Holmes Society; to Joyce Sackey and Sara Fazio, for being excellent partners as associate masters; and to Csilla Kiss, program coordinator for the Oliver Wendell Holmes Society, who always helps me meet my recommendation letter deadlines and is warm and welcoming to all who enter her office.

Thanks also to Antoinette Peters, PhD, for her help in integrating cross-cultural care into the tutorial through the use of "triggers" and for arranging for a mock tutorial, and to Roxana Llerena-Quinn, PhD, my knowledgeable collaborator on each of my workshops for the Association of American Medical Colleges' annual meetings on integrating cross-cultural care into preclinical science courses. I am extremely grateful to Vinod Nambudiri (MD and MBA, 2010), who as head of the student subcommittee of the Cross-Cultural Care Committee worked with me on the cases and triggers for integrating cross-cultural care into the tutorial. I thank Betty Crutcher, PhD, Marika McGrath, MA, and Martha Cesena, MD, for their terrific assistance on the cross-cultural care workshops for Harvard Medical School.

I am grateful to the following wonderful former fellows, residents, and students, who have worked with me in performing and writing up clinical and educational research projects, including, in chronological order, David Goran, MD, Felice Zwas, MD, Roger Sawhney, MD, Suzy Kim, MD, Jason Boch, DMSc, DMD, Andreas Gelrud, MD, Mita Goel, MD, John Branda, MD, Melissa Tukey, MD, and Laren Becker, MD, PhD.

Other terrific role models and teachers from the Office for Educational Development and the Academy include Elizabeth Armstrong, PhD, who shared her thoughts with me on being a medical educator in a personal interview in 2007 and who organized the superb Harvard Macy Institute Course on Leadership in 1999 that has influenced my subsequent career path and teaching style.

I appreciate the suggestions, recommendations, and tremendous teaching abilities of the members of the Gastrointestinal Advisory Committee, who have not been mentioned above, including, in alphabetical order, Alexander Carbo, MD, Darwin Conwell, MD, Kathleen Corey, MD, Laurie Fishman, MD,

John Kwon, MD, PhD, Richard Gardner, MD, Jeffrey Goldsmith, MD, Fiona Graeme-Cook, MB, BCh, Emily Hayden, MD, MA, HPE, Suma Magge, MD, Alan Moss, MD, Joseph Misdraji, MD, Daniel Pratt, MD, Marvin Ryou, MD, Elena Stoffel, MD, MPH, Matthew Turner, MD, and Menno Verhave, MD. I am also indebted to Anne Lyons, of the Newton, Massachusetts, Public School System, for sharing her superb teaching expertise and suggestions with the committee.

Family, friends, and colleagues who have given me valuable suggestions and opportunities include, in alphabetical order, Marci Christensen, RN, Sandra and Philip Gordon, Lisa Kamisher and Wayne Koch, MArch, Cynthia Kettyle, MD, and William Kettyle, MD, Annetta Kimball, MD, Har Kuan Kong, MS, Anne and Kenneth Lyons, Ann Louise Puopolo, BSN, RN, Mary Schaefer, RN, MEd, JD, and Eileen-Shields-West, MSFS, and John Robinson West, JD.

Thanks to Kitt Shaffer, MD, PhD, Melissa Upton, MD, and Ronald Rouse (of Harvard Medical School's Information Technology Department) for their help on our educational Web-based case project for the gastrointestinal pathophysiology course.

I am grateful to Joseph Martin, MD, PhD, former dean of Harvard Medical School, to the current dean of Harvard Medical School, Jeffrey Flier, MD, and to the dean of Medical Education, Jules Dienstag, MD, and Mary B. Clark, PhD, for their excellent support, advice, and suggestions.

My division chief of gastroenterology, J. Thomas LaMont, MD, and chair of medicine, Mark Zeidel, MD, at Beth Israel Deaconess Medical Center, enthusiastically support my teaching efforts.

Early in my academic career, I benefited from the expertise of the late Alexander Bearn, MD, chair of medicine at New York Hospital–Cornell Medical Center, who appointed me chief resident in medicine. Dr. Bearn gave me critical advice and guidance on writing research papers as well as giving a memorable lecture presentation. I am grateful to Sidney Cohen, MD, for being a role model for clinical attending on the gastroenterology service during my fellowship in gastroenterology at the University of Pennsylvania, where he was the chair, and for his subsequent support of my career advancement.

My thanks to Francis Giardiello, MD, MBA, and Robin Rutherford, MD, for joining me on an annual basis at Digestive Disease Week for the American Gastroenterological Association's "Tips for Poster Presenters." Thanks also to Jean-Pierre Raufman, MD, PhD, for his tireless efforts to improve the education of gastroenterologists through the Gastroenterology Teaching Project. I learned a great deal as a committee member from his management style and wisdom.

The other outstanding teachers, mentors, and assistants who have influenced the way I teach or helped me teach, are, in alphabetical order, Edward Achkar, MD, Donald Antonioli, MD, David Alpers, MD, Alfred Baker, MD, Jeremiah Barondess, MD, Elizabeth Boyd, PhD, Martha Cesena, MD, Sanjiv Chopra, MD, Jordan Cohen, MD, Carolyn Compton, MD, PhD, Julius Deren, MD, Joanne Donovan, MD, PhD, Franklin Epstein, MD, Christopher Fanta, MD, Francis Farraye, MD, MSc, Sara Fazio, MD, A. Stone Freedberg, MD, David Golan, MD, PhD, Joan Goldberg, MD, Harvey Goldman, MD, Raj Goyal, MD, Liza Green, Charles Hatem, MD, John Harrington, MD, Henry Heinemann, MD, Robert Heroux, Grace Huang, MD, Marshall Kaplan, MD, Jerome Kassirer, MD, B. Price Kerfoot, MD, EdM, George Kurland, MD, Robert Mayer, MD, James B. McGee, MD, Lori Newman, MEd, Donald Ostrow, MD, Elizabeth Peet, MA, James Patterson, MD, Orah Platt, MD, Edward Raffensperger, MD, Bernard Ransil, PhD, MD, Andrea Reid, MD, MPH, Suzanne Rose, MD, MSEd, Stanley Rosenberg, MD, Elihu Schimmel, MD, William B. Schwartz, MD, Richard Schwartzstein, MD, Roger Soloway, MD, Kathryn Stein, PhD, Charles Steinberg, MD, Joyce Sackey, MD, John Teall, PhD, Anjala Tess, MD, George Thibault, MD, Jerry Trier, MD, Steven Weinberger, MD, Louis Weinstein, MD, PhD, Lu Ann Wilkerson, EdD, Harland Winter, MD, and Gary Zuckerman, DO.

Librarians Nathan Norris, MLS, Diane Young, MLS, Henrietta Green, MLS, April Silver, MS, and Margo Coletti, MLS, AHIP, at the Agoos Medical Library of Beth Israel Deaconess Medical Center, Boston, and Julia Whelan, MS, AHIP, reference librarian of Francis A. Countway Library of Medicine, Boston, provided extraordinary help over the years with my questions about teaching and research projects. I am grateful to the Monroe C. Gutman Library at the Harvard Graduate School of Education and to the Derek Bok Center for Teaching and Learning at Harvard University for the many excellent references and teaching materials I found there.

Finally, I am grateful to Wendy A. Harris, medical editor of the Johns Hopkins University Press, for being an ideal editor and mentor throughout the book-writing process. Jacqueline C. Wehmueller, executive editor of the JHU Press, gave me positive feedback on my book proposal presentation at Dr. Julie Silver's excellent course on nonfiction medical book writing held in Boston in 2007. Emma L. Sovich, also at the Press, gave excellent help with the figures and permissions. I thank Barbara Lamb for her skill and care in the final editing of the book.

PART I

 Career Development

CHAPTER ONE

Why and How to Become a Successful Teacher

- 🌿 *What does successful mean?*
- 🌿 *Why do medical teaching assignments come with few, if any, instructions?*
- 🌿 *Why are certain teachers memorable?*
- 🌿 *How much time and effort will it take me to be like them?*
- 🌿 *Are there ground rules for success?*
- 🌿 *How do I translate some of my clinical abilities or research know-how to the educational realm?*

The Successful Medical Teacher

I define the successful medical teacher as someone who generates in the audience the desire to learn more; begins a conversation that students are anxious to continue; gives a framework for organizing material; distills complex concepts, making them simple to understand; leaves learners grateful; inspires others to teach; enjoys teaching; mentors other teachers; and believes and makes others believe that medicine is a great and proud profession.

Teaching is an exhilarating game of wits. I am constantly thinking of my next phrase, question, and gesture, adjusting and readjusting my tone, gaze, and intensity. I am in contact with my feelings about the audience's response to me, my response to them, and my next move.

Occasionally someone disparages great teachers by saying that they are "popular and fun to hear." However, while a few lecturers may be able to obtain high ratings from a "humorous and appealing talk," the great teacher has generally expended considerable effort in choosing the right visual images, making complex concepts clear, and providing a logical and well-reasoned approach to difficult medical problems. Great teachers are not "naturals." They are well-oiled machines accustomed to facing audiences with confidence because they have done their homework, listened to criticisms about past performances, reflected on and learned from their successes, and crafted and mastered a worthwhile presentation (Cole et al. 2004).

Teaching is one of the requirements for faculty members to hold positions at a medical school. Promotion boards on the investigator or clinician-teacher track at most medical schools look for evidence of evaluations indicating excellent medical teaching. Students, residents, fellows, and peers honor outstanding teachers, and teaching awards and prizes may recognize excellent teaching. These are some of the practical reasons to learn to be a great teacher. The personal reasons include satisfaction from doing a job well and intellectual stimulation from trying to clarify and distill medical and scientific concepts so that they are readily understood.

It is surprising that medical schools and hospitals do not instruct faculty members how to teach well (Bland et al. 1990). Over the years, I have tried to guess why recruiters and directors of teaching exercises hand out so few explicit instructions or tips on teaching. Perhaps it is because the directors themselves have not articulated on paper or out loud what works well and has made them successful as teachers. Alternatively, the course directors may feel that it is obvious how to teach well and think that tips or instructions are superfluous or even patronizing. They are there to be excellent head teachers, but not teachers of other teachers. Perhaps they are content to weed out the poor teachers, who drag down their course's ratings, and to hope for a better crop the following year. A darker interpretation is that some who know how to teach may not be eager to share this expertise in the competitive academic world, any more than some researchers share their antibodies or some clinicians their latest technical skill.

A separate roadblock to becoming a successful teacher is a faculty member's disinclination to do whatever it takes to achieve better ratings. Complacency, distain for constructive criticism, uncertainty about what to do and where to turn for help, or lack of time may make change too daunting (Skeff 2007). It is easier to accept the status quo of fair evaluations than to strive to be better.

Medicine creates a legacy for the next generation through great teaching, which is inspired and inspiring. Great teachers imbue us with a clear understanding and definition of scientific principles and show us the order, logic, beauty, and enticement of medicine. Continuing medical education courses, specialty meeting postgraduate courses, and research symposia vie for the best people to teach us new and cutting-edge science and medicine while we earn essential continuing medical education credits for licensure requirements. We go back to our practices or research with increased knowledge and motivation after contact with great teachers. How do they do it? Is it a natural or a finely honed talent? What are these dynamic and effective teachers doing, and how do they do it?

Developing into a Great Teacher

The simplest way to change your teaching style is to observe and copy great teachers. Medical teachers with excellent evaluations have deliberately acquired a skill set that frequently comes from observing other great teachers, talking to great teachers about the methods they use, and learning from faculty in other disciplines who teach well. Great medical teachers have worked hard to develop a superb fund of medical knowledge and have learned an organizational framework that helps learners understand complex concepts. They consistently approach each teaching assignment in an organized fashion.

Observe Great Teachers in Action

Videotaping of medical school preclinical courses makes it easy to observe great teachers. Ask your medical school curriculum support department if you can view tapes of the last three years' outstanding teacher awardees. If you do not know who these teachers are, ask your medical school librarian to locate their names from the teaching award announcements or awards' program. For clinical teachers, check the grand rounds listings for the past year. For research leaders, check the invited presenters' lecture schedules. Once you have located these teachers, go to their lectures or grand rounds. If you wish to see them in action in a tutorial, small group, or laboratory exercise, contact them directly and ask if you might observe. Explain that you are trying to improve your teaching skills and would appreciate the opportunity to learn from them. Few faculty members will deny you the privilege of watching them. Master teachers will notify their classes, tutorial students, seminar students, small groups, or laboratory students about your visit. They may wish you to come on certain days and not others, depending on the sensitivity of the discussion material. In clinical settings, some patients may refuse to have you observe a great clinician interacting with them. Usually, but not always, another date and time will be offered. Be grateful when you are permitted to watch. Always send a thank-you note to a teacher after you have observed a teaching session. If you subsequently improve as a teacher, let the teacher know that he or she was an integral part of your success.

Few faculty members take the time and make the effort to learn how to teach well. They will willingly watch a surgical procedure or an endoscopic technique, but they shy away from asking someone else in their department, hospital, or medical school if they can learn to teach better from them. Humility is useful to succeeding. Curiosity is essential. Why is that teacher getting applause? Is it what he or she is saying, or how he or she is saying it? Is it the visuals, the voice, the jokes, the asides, the organization, the content mastery, or the distillation of complex concepts? Is it the person's attitude toward teaching or toward the class? Until you understand what the person does and why the class responds to the person as it does, you can't change who you are as a teacher.

Go to the Medical Educators at Your Medical School to Learn Skills

I do not have an advanced degree in education. But in 1994, when I was appointed the sole director of the gastrointestinal pathophysiology course, I received education in curriculum design, assessment, leadership, and small-group direction from Miriam Wetzel, a PhD educator in Harvard Medical School's Office of Educational Development. In my quest to improve, I watched several great medical teachers at my institution on tape and in person in the late 1990s. I compared what they did with what I was doing. In 1999, I took the terrific Harvard Macy Institute Leadership Course, directed by Dr. Elizabeth Armstrong, who has created the highly successful Harvard Macy Program for Physician Educators at Harvard Medical School (Armstrong, Doyle, and Bennett 2003). I learned how to lead a discussion class from the Discussion Leadership Course given at Harvard University's Graduate School of Education by Dr. James Honan and the late Dr. Louis Barnes, in 2003.

Consider enrolling in a medical education course given by excellent and proven role models. In 2008, I enrolled in the Harvard Medical School and Beth Israel Deaconess Medical Center's first Annual Medical Education Course. During the course, I learned new techniques for improving my management of small groups, for outpatient office-based teaching, and for delivering a lecture.

Visit Business, Law, Government, and Public Policy Schools to Obtain New Ideas

If your backyard is an unappealing place to start your quest, go to a distant university or to another type of school to learn. In 2002, after listening to a lecture by Prof. David Garvin, of Harvard Business School, on the different case-based methods used by the medical, law, and business schools at Harvard University, I asked Professor Garvin for permission to watch his case-based discussion classes at Harvard Business School (Garvin 2003). I have gone back every year since then to watch vibrant classes. I have also watched classes at the John F. Kennedy School of Government, courtesy of Prof. Brian Mandell. The effort I have expended watching and listening to outstanding teachers has paid off with insights that have made me a stronger teacher. I altered my teaching style based on what I recognized as a more effective and successful style.

Altering Your Personal Teaching Style

Your personal teaching style is uniquely you as much as your clinical style is unmistakably you. Don't be stuck with a teaching style that is meeting resistance or less-than-optimal reviews. Learn how to replace learner resistance, scowls, glazed-over eyes, or blank stares with grateful smiles, interested questions, and the palpable relief of understanding at the end of your class, tutorial, attending rounds, grand rounds, physical diagnosis rounds, research data or journal club presentation (Palmer 2007). I have created simple guidelines for excellence in each of the above venues in the teaching-skills chapters of this book.

Ground Rules for Successful and Effective Teaching

Successful teachers are thoughtful, organized, and passionate about teaching. They care enormously, and it shows in the opportunities they seek for improved organizational skills, better faculty development, and mastery of content (fig. 1.1). In my quest to be a great teacher, I watched, listened, and tried a lot of ideas. Some worked and some didn't. From my successes and failures, I recognized that the first step in a teaching assignment is to decide what you are trying to accomplish by your lecture, small-group session, or laboratory exercise. Imagine your presentation and gauge the ratings you would give it. It helps to have a series of steps to reach the goal of excellent reviews

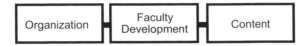

Figure 1.1. **Keys to Success**
Focus on intelligent but flexible organization, enthusiastic faculty development, and distillation of cutting-edge content for clarity. Be successful by distributing your energy equally among these three pillars of medical teaching.

(Whitaker 2004). A simple framework for each teaching assignment will save time. I created ground rules that make it much more likely that I will succeed than fail with any assignment I am given. These rules produce memorable teaching and grateful learners:

1. The objectives must be met full circle by the end of the session.
2. Master the content. Prepare intensively and extensively.
3. Develop a clear and logical flow to your presentation.
4. Explore the material using written questions.
5. Before you teach, visualize your future performance and desired evaluations. Adjust your presentation until you believe you will achieve your goals.
6. Create the right atmosphere for learning by skillfully managing group dynamics.
7. Reiterate important concepts throughout your presentation.
8. At the end of your presentation, solidify learning with a short closure summary using a visual schematic presenting clear illustrations of important concepts along with figures or tables demonstrating important take-home points.

These ground rules will be discussed in depth in succeeding chapters.

Use Your Clinical Skills and Research Expertise in Teaching

Some of the greatest teachers are also wonderful clinicians or world-renowned researchers. They use skills from clinical practice or research experiments to help them succeed as teachers. Communication skills are the major key to a successful clinical practice and grateful patients. These same skills will guarantee you a devoted following of students, residents, and fellows who rate you highly as a teacher who thinks out loud about decision making, underlying pathophysiology, evidence-based choices of therapy, and your philosophical approach to the patient. You are able to teach your secrets of successful medical care.

As a researcher, you have persistence in the face of adversity and flexibility to change course depending on the results. You question everything. Persistence will be invaluable in trying to find new ways to get through to your students. Flexibility will enable you to scrap teaching plans that are not working. Questioning everything will put you on the learner's side in trying to understand complex concepts.

I remember watching my first Harvard Business School discussion class in 2002. I came away in awe of Prof. David Garvin's preparation. He used a highly orchestrated and carefully prepared lesson plan (Barnes, Christensen, and Hansen 1994a, 1994b; Christensen 1991a, 1991b; Kasulis 1984). Each question to be asked was written down; during class, blackboards were skillfully filled; video-clips were carefully checked for a timely arrival during class. The take-away schematic was waiting as a handout after a rousing discussion (Greenwald 1991). My concept of teaching was forever changed by a glimpse of something better. My expectations for what medical education could be were raised with Professor Garvin's ninety-minute tour de force. I did not know how I was going to translate to medical school education what I had just seen, but I knew that this was what I wanted to do. I spent the next five years working out the translation of a business school case-based discussion class to a pathophysiology problem-based tutorial. The method was published in *Academic Medicine* in 2007 (Shields et al. 2007).

Recognize that changing body language or attitude or adding a new technique, a different method of preparation, or emphasis may lead to an extraordinary educational experience for you and your learners. Teachers who are striving to be better teachers look forward to the opportunity to teach differently and to get a better outcome, much as researchers live for the next experiment with the new reagent, the new strain of mouse, and the better outcome.

Perform Educational Research on Your Changes and Outcomes

As you strive to improve, you will constantly be changing your course, curriculum, or laboratory exercises. Make these changes count as career-building experiences by performing educational research projects to determine the outcome of your alterations. The changes will lead to more questions and more research. Submit an abstract to Research in Medical Education (RIME) at the Association of American Medical Colleges Annual Meeting or to your medical school's education day, or submit a paper to a journal interested in educational techniques, such as *Academic Medicine*. To perform the research experiment, obtain permission from your medical school's Institutional Review Board, write a proposal, and ask a statistician familiar with education who has access to learner and faculty evaluations for help with choosing and carrying out statistical analyses. Educational projects will become the subject of research papers that will launch your career as an academic teacher. See Chapter 14, "Bringing an Educational Research Project to Completion," for a step-by-step approach.

Is Teaching Worth the Effort?

When students, residents, and faculty greet me with a smile, a hello, or a thank you on the medical school or hospital campuses, it is frequently because I have taught them in class or in faculty development sessions. I enjoy the praise for a job well done (Stern et al. 2000). I also recognize that teaching medical students well and training faculty to teach better are significant parts of my medical legacy.

✂ TEACHING TIPS

1. The successful teacher stimulates students to want to learn more.
2. Don't expect explicit instructions on how to teach well.
3. Time, effort, and desire are necessary to change a teaching style.
4. Extensive preparation and content mastery, a logical plan with questions, and a summary of important points with a schematic are important elements of a successful teaching presentation.
5. The wish to constantly improve and the ability to learn from others are the marks of a great and successful teacher.
6. Make your teaching innovations your research projects; the research will launch and solidify your career as an academic medical teacher.

✂ TAKE-HOME POINTS

- To be a great teacher, copy great teachers.
- Spend time learning new teaching techniques at your institution and elsewhere; it will pay off.

- Develop a systematic approach; use ground rules to guarantee success.
- Use communication skills, questions, flexibility, and persistence to improve your teaching.
- Review, practice, and change your presentation until you believe you have achieved your ideal.

CHAPTER TWO

Personal Qualities of Successful Teachers

> 🦋 *What personal qualities are likely to give me the best evaluations of my teaching?*
> 🦋 *Does what I wear or how I look affect my evaluations?*
> 🦋 *Will I be perceived as a pushover if I am nice?*
> 🦋 *How do I handle students who are lacking in their preparation, participation, or attitude toward learning?*
> 🦋 *Is there a place for sarcasm?*
> 🦋 *Are there situations in which I should drop my nonjudgmental persona?*

Personal Qualities That Lead to Success

I do not want my learners to be distracted by my personality, my private thoughts, or my fears. When I watch a great play or movie, I want to relax and enjoy the actors' performances without knowing what they are thinking. The same is true for great teaching. Learners want to relax and gain understanding without distraction. I do the acting job necessary to get the result I want: learning. I aim for a performance that is smooth, upbeat, positive, and smart in content. I memorize my lines and practice my facial expressions, my mannerisms, and the tone of my voice in front of a mirror. I believe that I have an exciting message to deliver.

Cultivate an enthusiastic, curious, kind, nice, upbeat, positive, unflappable, even-tempered, sparkling, and nonjudgmental personality (Buchel and Edwards 2005; Cox and Swanson 2002; Elzubeir and Rizk 2001; Lawler, Chen, and Venso 2007; Markert 2001; Pinsky, Monson, and Irby 1998; Sutkin et al. 2008). These characteristics will encourage students to want to learn from you and be like you. Because wanting to learn is paramount to your accomplishing your goal as a teacher, it is wise to cultivate the personality traits of a winner. I am patient, open, friendly, pleasant, and willing to laugh at myself. I encourage suggestions to improve my performance. I anticipate students' needs. I try never to be arrogant, haughty, pompous, impatient, defensive, curt, annoyed, peevish, or adversarial. I avoid tentativeness. I maintain a stance that says I am on the students' side if they wish to learn. I will happily spend enormous time and effort helping them understand and achieve. I will lead them to new knowledge that they can make their own. See table 2.1 for the personal quali-

Table 2.1.   Personal Qualities of Teachers

A teacher is praised for being:

Enthusiastic	Positive	Available
Knowledgeable	Truthful	Approachable
Clear	Passionate	Gracious
Logical	Humble	Self-aware
Fair	Inspiring	Sensitive
Organized	Engaging	Responsible
Prepared	Flexible	A synthesizer
Thoughtful	Caring	A simplifier
Sparkling	Friendly	An advocate
Energetic	Nice	Respectful
Trustworthy	Pleasant	Polite
Reliable	Steadfast	Concerned
Confidence-building	Punctual	Empathetic
Warm	Understanding	Consistent
Supportive	Evenhanded	Humorous
Skillful	Even-tempered	Disciplined
Generous	Curious	Professional
Versatile	Unflappable	Nonthreatening
No-nonsense	Reassuring	Reflective
Creative	Nonjudgmental	

A teacher is criticized for being:

Unprepared	Petty	Dishonest
Aloof	Unavailable	Inconsistent
Disorganized	Confusing	Insensitive
Unclear	Incompetent	Irritable
Exhaustive	Cold	Sullen
Arrogant	Humorless	Unenthusiastic
Flippant	Pessimistic	Peevish
Illogical	A finger-pointer	Forgetful
Rigid	Obtuse	Unreliable
Tardy	Impatient	Tangential
Sarcastic	Pompous	Bombastic
Backbiting	Unhelpful	Insecure
Uncaring	Unaware of time	Officious
Defensive	Long-winded	Vindictive
Untruthful	Biased	

ties that lead to being a successful teacher and for the personal qualities that I have found may block learners from learning from me or another teacher.

To show that I care about each learner, I firmly shake hands with each student who comes into a small group. I look each person in the eye to show that he or she counts and to indicate that I wish to hear from him or her during the learning session. At the end of the preclinical course that I direct, I try to shake the hands of students and wish them well as they leave the auditorium after completing the proctored final exam.

Great teachers come in all sizes, shapes, voices, and dress. What is important is to be ready to teach. Students love to mimic and to caricature their teachers. A gravelly voice, a bow tie, a rolling suitcase (my signature), a bouffant hairdo, or a bushy beard will all be fodder for the annual student or resident spoof of teachers. Being ready to simplify and synthesize because you have mastered your content and are organized in your approach is far more important than what you wear or how you look. Learners are hungry for knowledge and are extremely pragmatic. It doesn't matter from whom the learning comes. Don't waste their time is the learner's cardinal request.

Being a nice teacher does not mean you are a pushover. You have rules and deadlines and will stick with them. But you are more effective in accomplishing your goals and in earning great evaluations if you are nice, pleasant, understanding, and when necessary, flexible.

I run late for many things, but not for a class or a teaching assignment. Being late sends the message that something else, other than teaching, is more important. This message is a bad beginning. If you are unavoidably late, apologize and try to stay after class to answer any questions. Don't be late again. Be early for the next class or session to show good faith and a mending of your ways.

Food is a useful icebreaker for discussion classes. Consider bringing fruit, cheese, crackers, nuts, muffins, or bagels as a way of creating a satisfied group that is ready to tackle a tough topic in a discussion.

Panic needs to be present before you teach, not when you teach. Panic pushes you to prepare sufficiently, but when the day and hour comes to teach, you must be calm and self-assured, like a baseball pitcher who dares not throw a wild pitch during a big game if he wishes to maintain his reputation.

Learners sense a teacher's fear of them. A teacher's fear will create a learning gulf that is hard to cross. I am fearful of failure before a teaching session, and this fear drives me to learn, study, practice, and polish my presentation to its fullest extent. If the evaluations are not excellent, I will have no regrets if I have done my best preparation. When the time comes to teach, I am ready and relaxed.

Everyone is equal in a class or small group. Don't court disaster by giving extra attention to the showoffs, the excellent students, and the hangers-on. Their attention may give you an ego boost, but you will be accused of favoritism behind your back. I recommend that you lavish as much attention on the quiet student whose eyes do not meet your gaze easily as on the student who is always asking terrific questions and lavishing praise on you. You will most likely find, as I have, that the students who are constantly at your side praising you and your teaching are frequently not the ones who will ace the exam. Rather, students whose names you barely remember will make you proud at exam time with how much they have learned from you.

I am not afraid to laugh at myself. It is great to be able to laugh when things go wrong, because so many things do go wrong. Fortunately, compared to clinical medicine, teaching is never a matter of life or death—just a matter of getting bad evaluations and less than optimal learning. To counteract bad evaluations, I am always open to suggestions about doing things differently. I am supportive of my students' desire to learn in the most effective and efficient manner possible.

Demonstrate your passion for teaching by having a tight organization to your course, class, and exercise. Be a reliable and responsible leader. Medical students, residents, fellows, and colleagues love organization in their teaching exercises. Your evaluations will be excellent if your organization facilitates smooth sailing.

Professionalism Is Important

Keep your negative feelings about mishaps and glitches in check. Learners want a friendly, accepting, peaceful atmosphere. They want to relax, focus, and concentrate. If you have a complaint about your media person, your administrator, your colleague, your nurse, a student, keep it to yourself. No one who is trying to learn from you wants to hear complaints, fuming, and frustration. Address and fix problems behind the scenes. It is your job to make things happen correctly by checking and rechecking. Despite your best efforts, when a glitch occurs, such as handouts, syllabus, evaluations not being ready or available for your class or group, face the music with "the buck stops here" approach and apologize to the class. Keep the behind-the-scenes commotion behind the scenes. Venting may make you feel better, but you have likely dropped your ratings into the sub-basement. My husband will hear all about my frustrations the evening of my latest teaching disaster, but my students will not. Choose someone you can trust who is outside the fray and go over your disappointments with that person, not the class.

Handling Subpar Performances

You should not vent to the class as a whole about their lackluster performance if you want the students who have been doing their work quietly and effectively to respect you. These students will be distressed at your not seeing the conscientious efforts they are making. Do not lump good learners with the subpar group, as this will only anger both sets of students. Instead of a rant against the whole group, begin focusing your energies on those who are listening and trying to learn. Take aside disinterested, disenchanted students, interns, residents, and fellows. What you will find out from these problem learners in a one-on-one conference is usually helpful. Frequently, the learners' performance has been poor due to personal and family stresses or to their own medical problems. Don't burden with the lackluster label the learners who have heard your directions and are trying hard to please you. You may poison the well of good will you have. A successful teacher takes the high road.

Maintaining a Nonjudgmental Mien in a Difficult Situation

Be nonjudgmental in your attitude toward learners. This means being open to other points of view and opinions. It means being welcoming. It does not mean being insensitive, blind, or "Pollyanna-like" to what is happening in your classroom, rounds, or small group. I have occasionally had to step outside my nonjudgmental mien when I believe the entire group's ability to learn is being hurt by a student's or my own gesture, remark, or body language. At these times, I'll state that I am stepping out of my teaching persona to try to right a wrong or to give breathing room for an honest discussion of what has just occurred and how I feel about it. I'll call for a time out. I try to carefully gauge my words and tone of voice to capture what I feel in a dispassionate manner. I may ask for help from the class to recognize and heal the rift that is developing. I will weigh in with my own judgment to try to clarify and diffuse a difficult situation.

A recent example of my stepping outside a nonjudgmental stance occurred when, for the first time in fifteen years of tutoring, a student brought a laptop to the nine-person tutorial. When I saw the laptop opened up, I asked the student to put it away because I felt it would distract me and the other students if the student were to begin typing during a discussion course in which probing questions may be addressed to each student. The questions and answers create a complex flow of fast-paced discussion focused on understanding pathophysiologic concepts. The student with the laptop was clearly offended and annoyed by my request. The rest of the group looked uncomfortable. Although the student put the laptop away, I was aware that I was being viewed as arbitrary and inflexible. After polling a number of students in different years about the use of laptops in a discussion class or tutorial that afternoon, I called the student late that evening to apologize for being so brusque in my request that he not use the laptop in the tutorial. The student accepted the apology and said he was pleased that I had called. At the next tutorial, I started with a brief discussion of my actions and my regret at being arbitrary and curt in handling the situation, but I reiterated my wish that students not use laptops in the tutorial. The unpleasant situation was diffused somewhat, and the group functioned reasonably well after the problem had been aired.

Letting down your nonjudgmental face is risky but may be the right thing to do when a wrong has occurred on your watch. Trying to fix it later is often too late. The damage is done to your class and to your creditability as a respected teacher. "Strike while the iron is hot" is an apt proverb for damage control in teaching. Don't let hurt or misunderstandings fester in your class or group. Diffuse them quickly.

Do Sarcasm, Innuendo, or Cutting Remarks Have a Role?

You are not running for a political office against an opponent. In politics, sarcasm, innuendo, and cutting or biting remarks are taken as signs of intelligent repartee. You are trying to lead tired, poorly paid physicians or jaded students to learn important concepts. Leave sarcasm and biting comments at the door. Instead, cultivate an atmosphere of mutual respect, admiration, honesty, and collegiality by speaking with a silver rather than a forked tongue. You will get the action that you want: learning, not rebellion.

What Does Unflappable Mean?

Be unflappable; this means that the show goes on no matter what. Two years ago, I was sitting in the front row of the auditorium listening to the lecture entitled "Pancreas" when a student tripped while coming into the lecture hall late. Her drink dropped to the floor, sending a pile of yogurt up into the air. The round blob of yogurt landed on the top of my head. I would have liked to take the yogurt off the top of my head but knew that this would disturb the whole class. Instead, I turned around and smiled at the class, letting them know that I knew how silly I looked. I waited until the hour lecture was over to remove the yogurt from my hair. A student later labeled my behavior as "unflappable."

Qualities That Count

I want an even-tempered, even-handed, energetic, enthusiastic person with a sense of humor to teach me. Having all the right personality characteristics will not make up for weak content or poor organization. Nor will they take away the anger of your students if your overly long presentation forces them to miss their coffee break or be late for their next class. Focus first on knowing what you want to get across, then on your organization, your lesson plan, your teaching skills, and finally on your timing. If you add in a pleasant, nice, kind, enthusiastic personality, you have an unbeatable combination. What learner could want more?

The Most Important Quality

The most important quality of a successful teacher is the same quality I would put as my first choice for being a successful physician: respect. If you have respect for the learner, it will show in your careful preparations, your engagement of the learner with questions, your modulation of the dominant student to bring in the quiet student, your painstaking distillation of all you wish the learner to know, your thoughtful summary, and your creative "take-away."

You will start on time to stay on time; your session and handouts will be well organized, streamlined, and focused on learning. Every precious moment of the learner's time will be carefully orchestrated toward learning. Repetition, the mother of learning, will be embraced, not derided. Teaching the same concept from multiple angles, until the concept is clear, will be routine.

✌ TAKE-HOME POINTS

- Learning is best done in a pleasant atmosphere; create this atmosphere.
- Leave favoritism out of teaching.
- Your nonjudgmental mien may need to be suspended to right a wrong.
- Forget sarcasm; speak with a silver tongue.
- Cultivate your tone of voice and facial expressions to be upbeat and positive.
- Be unflappable, but not unaware.
- Never let problems fester; fix them promptly.
- Panic before, never during a teaching session.
- Let fear drive your preparation, never your presentation.

CHAPTER THREE

How to Succeed as a Medical Educator

    What is the difference between a medical teacher and a medical educator?

    What types of skills are expected of an educator?

    How do I get trained in teaching skills?

    What are my job prospects?

    What are some obstacles to success?

    What are the rewards?

A Medical Educator: Definition, Skills, and Training

The word *doctor* comes from the Latin word *docere*, which means to teach. Consequently, all doctors are teachers. Doctors, though, may not have formal training in teaching. A medical educator is defined as one who is trained in teaching or is a specialist in the theory and practice of education. A medical educator is engaged in creating, developing, leading, and researching in order to change and improve medical education. Hesketh et al. (2001) devised a framework for developing excellence as a clinical educator that names twelve tasks the educator should be able to do, such as competently teach large and small groups; teach in a clinical setting; plan, learn, and evaluate courses; and undertake research in education.

A medical educator is trained in a core set of academic skills. Dr. Elizabeth Armstrong, director of the Harvard Macy Institute (Friedrich 2002), organized these skills into five different areas: (1) teaching and learning, (2) curriculum design, (3) assessment, (4) leadership, and (5) information technology. These are discussed in subsequent chapters.

As an educator, you will share your expertise and skills, mentor and train others, create new curricula, and plan for the present and future of medical education using strong leadership and organizational skills.

Most physicians who decide to become medical educators do so because they were exposed to great teachers in the preclinical classroom, on attending rounds, at grand rounds, or at a specialty conference. The intellectual vigor, enthusiasm, energy, and superb speaking ability of these teaching giants make them wonderful and memorable role models to emulate. Mentors, who are defined as people of advanced rank or experience who guide, teach, and develop a newcomer to the profession, may also be admired teachers from high school, college, medical school, recognized educational leaders, hospital attending physicians, PhD or EdD educators, interdepartmental teaching icons, chairs of departments, or deans. The key characteristic of the teacher-mentor is the willingness to share knowledge, teaching "secrets," philosophy, and contacts. Multiple mentors can help with different skills and should be cultivated. It is uncommon to find one person who is able to mentor all skills needed. Zerzan et al. (2009) created a checklist to help mentees establish successful mentoring relationships. Mentors are generally the ones to recommend the medical educator for opportunities for increased visibility and contacts, including education committees, invited conferences, speaking engagements, book chapters, and research projects.

Training in educational methods is important for acceptance as a potential leader in the medical education field. Several options exist, including doing a chief residency, which has been shown to be positively correlated with being considered an excellent attending-physician role model at a teaching hospital (Wright et al. 1998), obtaining a master's or PhD degree in education, doing a fellowship in medical education, taking medical education courses or residential and on-line courses, and watching videotapes of excellent teachers. A chief resident position offers basic training in medical administrative, organizational, and teaching skills. In addition, the chief residency position, which I held at New York Hospital–Cornell Medical Center, gave me tremendous experience in people skills and managing group dynamics. The chief resident position also taught me how to initiate an educational activity, overcome all obstacles to making the dream a reality, get buy-in from crucial faculty and residents to get a good start, critically reflect on the maiden voyage of the new educational activity, and write down for posterity what should be changed or kept the same to make it a successful ongoing activity.

Formal training in education may be advisable to ensure acceptance and career success. Several universities, such as the University of Illinois at Chicago (www.uic.edu/com/mcme), Stanford University (http://sfdc.stanford.edu/progct), the University of California at Los Angeles (http://dgsom.health sciences.ucla.edu/education/md/joint-programs), the University of Michigan (www.med.umich.edu/meded/programs/mesp.htm), and the University of Dundee, in Scotland (c.m.e.@dundee.ac.uk), offer master's programs in medical education or health education. The master's degree in health education from the University of Illinois may be obtained in a flexible on-line curriculum or as a residential program. This is also true for the master's degree from the University of Dundee. A master's degree or a doctorate in education is useful, provided that the focus is on adult rather than childhood learning.

Medical education courses sponsored for junior and senior faculty by the Harvard Macy Institute include doing an approved project to be brought back to the participant's medical school. The Harvard Macy Institute (www.harvard macy.org) provides valuable opportunities to learn new methods and skills. Yearlong fellowships in medical education are offered for faculty at Stanford University and through the Rabkin Fellowship in Medical Education at Boston's Beth Israel Deaconess Medical Center's Shapiro Institute for Education and Research (http://bidmc.org/medicaleducation). Other ways to learn are to observe or audit classes at schools of education, business, law, or government, where the teaching methods may be different but are adaptable to medical education. Videotapes of great lecturers and small-group leaders are helpful for defining what the great teacher does to engage the audience in learning.

Finally, on-the-job training is an acceptable way to learn the ropes of curriculum creation and faculty development as well as the tools of evaluation and assessment. A mentor who has a master's, a PhD, or a doctorate in education (EdD) is a valuable resource.

Navigating the Academic Environment

Medical educators traditionally focus on one specific group, such as medical students, residents, fellows, or their peer group, for the majority of their teaching and education efforts. My primary focus is on two groups: medical students and gastroenterology fellows. Years ago, I realized that I enjoyed teaching pathophysiology more than clinical medicine. The natural consequence of my enjoyment of teaching pathophysiology is my focus on medical students and specialty fellows rather than on clinical residents, because the need to learn pathophysiology is largely a preclinical requirement for passing the United States Medical Licensing Examination (USMLE), Step 1 and Step 2, and a requirement for the specialty boards. The USMLE is developed and managed by the National Board of Medical Examiners (NBME). In 2002, I established a yearly teaching fellow position for a gastroenterology fellow to learn the basics of tutoring, small-group teaching, curriculum creation, faculty development, evaluation, assessment, and central aspects of study design for research in medical education.

Colleagues of mine have focused their careers on resident, fellow, or peer-group teaching, on continuing medical education activities (CME), or on teaching patients and the community at large. Some educators are able to successfully teach in all areas. Medical educators teach and lead educational activities in medical schools, hospitals, university settings, CME postgraduate courses, community outreach programs, and at international conferences and at other medical schools. Educators may focus their efforts on the creation of Web-based educational material, such as Dr. Peter Kelsey has done with the DAVE Project (http://dave1.mgh.harvard.edu), Dr. James B. McGee has done with the American Gastroenterological Association's Web-based teaching modules (www.gastro.org; go to Education and Training, then to Online Education and CME), and Dr. B. Price Kerfoot, with Spaced Education, an on-line teaching tool (www.spaceded.com).

Fellows and junior faculty are frequently asked to be in charge of one or more teaching conferences at the hospital or to supervise medical students or residents who require teaching, mentoring, and evaluations. Acceptance of these types of teaching assignments is a good way to begin to learn the organizational and people-management skills necessary to direct a preclinical or clinical course or CME activity. Doing the best job possible without fuss or complaints and showing consistent excellence in teaching, organizational abilities, and skillful personnel leadership often leads to recognition and larger teaching assignments.

It is helpful to improve career opportunities and gain visibility by winning annual teaching awards. Another way to win recognition is to be named to a teaching fellowship that enhances teaching skills, such as the fellowships in medical education available at:

1. Stanford University, through Dr. Kelly Skeff and the Stanford Faculty Development Center for Medical Teachers, where faculty interested in improving clinical teaching skills can apply to the program for a one-month intensive course under the direction of Dr. Skeff and Dr. Stratos (http://sfdc.stanford.edu); contact Georgette A. Stratos, PhD, Stanford Faculty Development Center, 700 Welch Road, Suite 310B, Palo Alto, CA 94304-1809, phone: 650 725-8802, fax: 650 725-1675).

2. The University of Michigan's Medical Education Scholars Program, a ten-month program designed to develop leaders in health science education. Dr. Stanley J. Hamstra (shamstra@umich.edu) is the director of the Department of Medical Education, which administers the annual program. The program brochure is available at www.med.umich.edu/meded/programs/mesp.htm.

3. Beth Israel Deaconess Medical Center and Harvard Medical School's Rabkin Fellowship in Medical Education is open to all faculty with a primary appointment at Harvard Medical School and is a year long opportunity to undertake a scholarly research project or an educational project in the applicant's area of interest.

4. The University of Illinois, Chicago, College of Medicine Short-Term Fellowships, which accept applicants from around the country for a three-month project of the applicant's choice. Educational research development and study activities are tailored to address each project goal. Information about these fellowships can be accessed from the Department of Medical Education's home page, at http://cores33 webs.mede.uic.edu/dme/warp/dme_search.asp.

5. The Harvard Macy Institute offers in-depth one-week programs for Leading Innovations in Health Care and Education and A Systems Approach to Assessment in Health Science Education. Participants come from around the country for these intensive medical education programs (harvard_macy@hms.harvard.edu). Applicants apply months ahead for these programs.

6. The University of Washington's Teaching Scholars Program accepts qualified individuals from the school of medicine, dentistry, social work, pharmacy, and nursing, as well as foreign scholars who are studying at the University of Washington, for a one-year program that promotes innovation and educational leadership (contact Lynne Robins, PhD, Director, Teaching Scholars Program, at lynner@u.washington.edu) (Robins, Ambrozy, and Pinsky 2006).

Designing educational research projects and writing proposals for grant funding may lead to publications, which are essential to eventual promotion on the teacher-clinician track. Medical educators are usually involved in both clinical and research activities in addition to medical education to completely cover the cost of their salaries. Advising and mentoring medical students, residents, and fellows is an additional way to obtain income from medical schools and hospitals.

Opportunities for Research, Publication, and Leadership

The field of medical education is full of opportunities for research. Each change in curriculum or faculty development lends itself to evaluation and assessment with careful research-study design. Evaluation of changes by faculty and students is generally by pre- and postintervention questionnaires, which require approval by the medical school's institutional review board. Assessment generally uses a quantitative measure, such as the objective structured clinical examination (OSCE) or USMLE scores. Clinical reviews of disease processes, book chapters, and writing for the lay public are recognized on the teacher-clinician track and solidify the case for promotion. Demonstration of leadership and successful innovation in educational activities are keys to promotion. Look for opportunities to lead and create educational activities at the local, national, and international levels, whether through organizing a new course, developing a grant proposal involving input from educators at different medical schools, bringing an educational symposium to completion, or directing or co-directing a postgraduate course.

Best Evidence in Medical Education

As you are performing research in the field of medical education, you will note the paucity of randomized controlled trials for educational innovations. Many studies use historical controls or observational control groups. Best Evidence in Medical Education (BEME) Collaboration is a group supported by the Association for Medical Education in Europe (AMEE), which is an international association for medical education (amee@dundee.ac.uk). BEME is committed to the promotion of the best evidence in medical education through the dissemination of information that permits educators to make decisions on the best evidence available and to the production of thoughtful and well-researched reviews of broad topics in medical education. Their Web site (www.BEMEcollaboration.org) provides ten published systematic review guides on diverse medical education subjects as free downloads.

Funding and Remuneration for the Medical Educator

Small grants are readily obtainable from medical schools and foundations interested in improving medical education. Chairs of departments much appreciate a small grant that pays a fraction of salary for you to create new curriculum. Salaries are lower for the medical educator than the clinician, but the educator must still be alert to garnering salary from the medical school, the resident or fellowship program, or continuing medical education activities in order to meet his or her obligations to bring salary or funds for teaching to whatever department he or she is affiliated with. Be aware that discrepancies may exist at your medical school and hospital in the salaries given to those who teach in preclinical and clinical medical student programs and those who administer the preclinical or clinical programs. In addition, physicians who direct residency or fellowship programs may be given considerably different salaries from preclinical course directors.

Make no assumptions about your salary compensation for teaching activities. If a salary stipend is important to you or to your chair, ask at the outset how much you will be paid for your efforts. Will you be paid by the hour for face-to-face teaching? Will you be paid a flat or fixed rate for running a clerkship, a course, or a principal clinical experience that is longitudinal? How much salary will you be paid for being a course director, a residency or a fellowship director? Is it negotiable? Will it cover the numerous hours you put into making the program a stellar one? Will the salary be increased if you do well? Forewarned is forearmed. Only if you ask directly about the compensation package you will receive, and what it is based on, will you know the answers to these questions.

In 1994, when I was appointed sole director of the gastrointestinal pathophysiology course, I was so happy that I never asked how much salary I was going to receive for running the three-week-long course. I was basking in the glow of creating new teaching materials and exercises, oblivious to the fact that there was no specific salary, but only a small stipend paid to my department chair, for my being a preclinical course director at the medical school. Had I asked and found out that no specific salary was going to be paid to my department to offset the hours I spent in preparation and teaching time, I may have been discouraged from pursuing what I enjoyed so much. I cannot second-guess my decision sixteen years later, when I have had so much fun and such a memorable and satisfying experience being a course director. Instead, my history has taught me to recommend that others ask up-front how much salary, if any, they will be given for their efforts. Bring this defined monetary figure to a discussion with your chair, and weigh the chair's response in your decision to accept, reject, or negotiate a better salary for the educational leadership position you have been offered.

Opportunities for Women and Minorities

Medical education provides an excellent career opportunity for both women and minorities to consider. Many of the prominent figures in the field are women. However, promotion to full professor on the teacher-clinician track may pose difficulties for women who have small children, given the need for traveling to speaking engagements at the national or international levels and the pressure to publish to rise to the rank of full professor.

Helpful Organizations for Medical Educators

American College of Physicians (ACP) (www.acponline.org). The organization holds an annual meeting with leadership courses and internal medicine updates in key areas. In addition, the ACP puts out the MKSAP review materials, publishes the *Annals of Internal Medicine,* and sponsors internal medicine board review courses.

American Gastroenterological Association Institute (AGA) (www.gastro .org). The AGA has an active Committee on Education, a Committee on Web-Based Education, and a Committee on Program Evaluation, as well as educational AGA Institute publications for laypeople and for specialists. Journals published by the association are *Gastroenterology* and *Clinical Gastroenterology and Hepatology.*

Association of American Medical Colleges (AAMC) (www.aamc.org). The organization holds an annual meeting with sessions on research in medical education, gives courses to improve educational skills, and has geographic groups on educational affairs. The AAMC publishes *Academic Medicine,* an excellent source of innovations in medical education.

Association for the Study of Medical Education (ASME) (info@asme.org .uk). Located in Edinburgh, Scotland, the association publishes the monthly journal *Medical Education* and the quarterly journal *Clinical Teacher.*

Association for Surgical Education (www.surgicaleducation.com). This association promotes, recognizes, and rewards excellence, innovation, and scholarship in surgical education. It helps develop innovative teaching aids, programs, and effective surgical interventions and designs faculty development programs for surgical education.

Harvard Macy Institute (harvard_macy@hms.harvard.edu). The institute offers medical education and leadership courses that are beneficial at all levels of academic medicine.

International Association of Medical Science Educators (IAMSE) (www .iamse.org/contact.htm). The annual meeting of this organization is designed for all those who teach and lead curricula in medicine. The aim is to improve teaching of both normal structure/function and pathophysiology, and both basic science and clinical education.

International Society of Pathophysiology (ISP) (email: xj.arthur@gmail .com). The ISP is a nongovernmental, nonprofit organization uniting specialists of experimental physiology, clinical medicine, and modern biology who work on the problems of human and animal pathophysiology. Better teaching of pathophysiology is a major goal.

Society of Academic Emergency Medicine (SAEM) (saem@saem.org). This society's mission is to improve and advance research and education in the field of emergency medicine. The society publishes *Academic Emergency Medicine.*

Society of General Internal Medicine (SGIM) (www.sgim.org). The Education Committee devises and implements plans to address the needs of medical educators, including developing strategies for improving the level of teaching competencies and models to evaluate and reward excellence in teaching and scholarship. Its annual meeting has a focus on improving medical education. The society publishes the *Journal of General Internal Medicine,* with a yearly education update.

Society of Teachers of Family Medicine (www.stfm.org). This society's annual predoctoral education conference for family medicine educators helps participants stay abreast of new research, cutting-edge technologies, and best practices.

Many other specialty organizations have education programs that offer terrific opportunities for advancement in the specialty field and as a medical teacher or educator. Search online for the specialty you are invested in, and organizations that have educational activities will appear. Contact these organizations or attend a workshop or meeting that advertises improving teaching skills.

Career Prospects

The career prospects for medical educators are numerous and bright, but to succeed, you must acquire a set of teaching skills. Formal training is useful for

Table 3.1.   Obstacles and Rewards for Medical Educators

Obstacles

   Need for protected time to create materials, develop programs, and do research
     projects

   Requirement for coverage of clinical activities during teaching assignments

   Awards as well as publications generally needed for promotion

   Compensation usually not competitive or commensurate with the salary a clinician
     would receive for a similar number of hours

Rewards

   Long career with no upper age limit

   Burgeoning field

   Room for new ideas

   Improved chances for promotion in recent years

   Satisfaction from creation of enjoyable, effective, and efficient learning

   Helping other physicians develop into better medical teachers

   Lifelong learning

advancement, recognition, and acceptance. Mentors who encourage, guide, share expertise, and recommend the educator for teaching assignments and promotions are essential. Recognize that educators also support their salaries by being clinicians and researchers. Promotion usually requires both teaching awards and educational publications. The rewards for being a medical educator are many, and include helping others become better teachers.

Table 3.1 lists obstacles and rewards for medical educators.

✂ TEACHING TIPS

1. Choose the learner type you like best and feel most comfortable with for the majority of your teaching; become an expert at this level of teaching.

2. Avail yourself of opportunities to obtain grants and do educational research; the payoff will be a promotion.

3. Don't be afraid to start at the bottom and work your way up the teaching ladder.

4. Salaries will be lower, but satisfaction may be higher with a career focus in education.

5. Ask up-front about salary compensation for your teaching; negotiation may be possible.

✂ TAKE-HOME POINTS

- **To get ahead, get trained.**
- **Use multiple mentors; each will shine at a different skill.**
- **Small teaching responsibilities done well lead to big teaching responsibilities.**
- **Get coverage of your clinical duties during teaching assignments or risk doing poorly at both.**

PART II

 Teaching Skills

CHAPTER FOUR

A Framework for Successful Teaching

- *How do I prepare for a teaching presentation?*
- *What steps should I take to receive excellent learner evaluations?*
- *Are there foolproof ways for engaging students/learners?*
- *What are common mistakes in teaching, and how can I avoid them?*
- *Do I need to pay attention to each and every criticism of my teaching?*

A Mindset for Successful Teaching

Recently, a third-year medical student doing her core clerkship in surgery fell in step with me as I walked from one hospital building to another. She said that she wanted to thank me for helping her, and her entire class, understand gastrointestinal pathophysiology. I told her how much I appreciated her comments. Inwardly, I hoped she would praise specific parts of the course, such as its structure and organization, energetic faculty, small-group breakout sessions, or tutorials, so I would know in what areas I had succeeded. Instead, she said that I obviously cared about whether students learned the material. In her view, my caring about students' learning was my greatest strength, which set me apart from other preclinical teachers. I admit disappointment. But, I also realized that caring about learner satisfaction is a wonderful character trait to nurture in future medical teachers and in oneself.

To care, you need to forget that you are paid very little or not at all. You need to forget that going up for promotion on the teacher-clinician ladder is fraught with difficulties, that getting published in medical education journals is not easy, and that most physicians take for granted what you do as a teacher and view medical teaching as a "soft" side of medicine. If you let these realities intrude on your idealism, you will not care enough to be innovative in the face of adversity, to persist in trying to improve your teaching, and to go the extra mile to make your teaching clear and instructive.

When I teach, I keep in my mind's eye the parents of the students. Are the parents getting their money's worth for their son's or daughter's medical education? Over vacation periods, will students be badmouthing medical school teaching or praising it? Will students tell their parents that teaching in medical school is a letdown after the inspirational college teaching they had? Thinking as a parent makes me care about medical school teaching and about doing it well.

Follow a Framework

I use a five-step framework for teaching successful educational exercises (table 4.1), no matter what the particular teaching assignment may be. This framework is an essential tool to teach memorable learning sessions and is applicable to being a tutor, small-group leader, lecturer, workshop leader, teaching attending on the clinical services, or teacher of physical diagnosis. The framework consists of five simple steps: (1) visualization, with the creation of transparent objectives; (2) intensive preparation to learn current knowledge, evidence for the objectives, and the design of questions to guide exploration of the material; (3) distillation of important concepts in an upbeat presentation, including a summary, preferably with a schematic; (4) concrete realizations of how the presentation went; and (5) self-reflection, leading to refinement and changes of future teaching assignments.

Step 1. Visualization

What do I mean by visualization? Each weekend, you probably visualize your errand route to the post office, bank, grocery store, hardware store, or dry cleaner to save gas, steps, and time. Visualizing your teaching session is similar in that you outline in your head your path, your presentation, and your likely results. To visualize your performance, flash forward to the day of teaching. How will you look, what will you wear? What will your tone be, and how will you sound? How will the audience respond to you, to your slides, facial expressions, jokes, blackboard or chalk talk? Will they feel they learned something new or valuable? Will the audience enjoy the process of learning and be energized?

Visualizing is not only a measure of how well the talk or presentation will be received but also a way of anticipating mistakes and errors. Somewhat like Charles Dickens's Ebenezer Scrooge in *A Christmas Carol*, you need to see into the future to correct the present. Visualizing means allowing yourself to day-

Table 4.1. Five Simple Steps for Teaching Successful Educational Exercises

---

Visualization: How will I do it?

Preparation: What do I want to teach?

Presentation: How will I teach it?

Realizations and Reflection: How did it go from the learners' perspective and from my perspective?

Refinement: What should I do differently next time to be more effective and to obtain better evaluations?

---

dream about how your session will go. You may then anticipate that you will be unprepared because there is too much on your calendar to prepare properly. The best option may be to immediately decline the teaching invitation in favor of another date, for which you can prepare, or to cancel things that are in conflict with your preparation. You may anticipate that the field you are asked to speak on is not your specific interest but your colleague's, and you may be happy to recommend that the talk be turned over to him or her. You may see yourself giving a brilliant lecture with your new research data. You may anticipate an excellent small-group learning experience as long as you spend the time to organize the material, outline your goals and objectives, and achieve them.

When you anticipate and preview your performance, will you hear applause and see admiring looks of approval or will you see glazed-over or somber looks on your learners' faces? Will there be the excitement of learning in the room or flatness and dullness? Will many learners in the front rows be sleeping? Are you confident, calm? Do you sound knowledgeable, approachable, and pleasant? Do you see yourself becoming nervous and uneasy because you lack good command of your material? Do you worry that you will not have practiced the talk sufficiently, that the slide presentation will not project, or that you cannot answer the questions the audience asks? Are you late to your own presentation because you failed to cancel your last clinic patients, find accurate directions, or test the route to your teaching venue to see how long it would take to get there in rush-hour traffic? Is your beeper going off during your presentation because you did not sign it out? Are you trying to squeeze forty slides into a twenty-minute time slot, one of the commonest mistakes? Are you apologizing for dense-data slides, crammed with rows of numbers too small to be seen from the back rows?

An organized framework is an essential tool for the teacher to teach a memorable and active learning session, no matter what the venue. Design transparent objectives that become a teaching plan and framework for all your anticipated major points. Just as on a Saturday errand trip, you have your priorities concerning the stores you must visit before arriving home and those that can wait; you need a "must-cover list" of objectives. How will you prioritize the objectives? Will the objectives be clear to the audience? How will you make them clear? Will you use slides, a flip chart, a handout, or just state the objectives before you start? Will you cover all your objectives? See chapter 5 for a description of the types of objectives.

Step 2. Preparation

A new teaching assignment results in short-changing something or someone else. The new assignment, if it is done well, will negatively affect your already-crowded schedule. Other deadlines may not be met. When you are asked to teach, think carefully. Weigh the pros and cons before you say yes. Does doing a great job of teaching mean that other important projects will go to seed? What are the consequences of doing a poor job? Is the upheaval in your schedule worth the honor of the assignment? Accept teaching assignments only if you have the time to do a good job. Otherwise beg off, if possible, until you can free up time to prepare. This will not be the last teaching assignment you are asked to accept.

If you accept the assignment, prepare in several ways. First, do a recent literature search using PubMed and/or Paper Chase and other search engines. Ask your hospital or university medical librarian to obtain articles not available on the digital library or through interlibrary loan. The day of your presentation, you do not want to hear, "What do you think of the recent or classic journal article?" when you have not read this article or, worse yet, are unaware of its existence. Second, find classic articles in the field by checking the bibliography of monographs and review articles. Use your objectives as a guide. As you read, you may realize that your objectives need to change to include a new point or to exclude what is now an outmoded or irrelevant point.

If you are the invited expert in the field, why bother to read and prepare? You should prepare so that you are not guilty of delivering a "canned" talk. Some "canned" talks are outstanding, but some sound tired, recycled, stale, and unexciting. Don't skimp on preparation just because you have given the lecture before or are an expert. Reading the latest literature, even if you are a significant writer of that literature, injects energy and freshness into your talk or discussion group. Keep abreast of the *New York Times* science or medicine sections or your local newspaper's science and medicine news. Newspapers generally carry the latest controversies and summaries of the top journal findings on a weekly basis. Check the literature and the newspapers the day before your talk and the day of your talk. An important article or item that could change your talk's premise and conclusions may have quietly slipped into the news or the literature.

As you read, begin to make an outline of your introduction, the body of your talk, the questions you will use to explore controversial areas and cover the objectives, key points you wish to reiterate, and the summary. What is the level of your learner group? Are they first-year medical and dental students or first-year residents, subspecialty fellows, clinical attending physicians, full-time practitioners, or basic researchers? Is your talk at the end or the beginning of the day? Is the talk between the coffee break and a popular lecturer? Is the time allotted too short? Logically organizing your talk is the most important way of ensuring that the audience will follow your points. The audience wants to relax and enjoy the discovery of new knowledge packaged in a readily graspable format. Logical progression underlies a great teaching session.

Start to obtain your visuals from the articles you read, your own image archives, research data tables, figures, and explanatory diagrams. In this age of nonstop colorful visual displays on the Internet, it is important to have visual aids that carry the content message while being visually appealing. Review each of your handouts, slides, and syllabi for their utility and attractiveness. Make sure you know how each picture or word slide advances the coherence of your presentation. During your practice phase, you will usually need to delete some of your visuals to stay within the time frame.

Every medical learner enjoys real-life cases that emphasize the dos and don'ts and the vagaries of diagnosis and treatment in medicine. You may have fabulous case material to use if, over the years, you have written down each patient's name, medical record number, and major findings after seeing him or her in your clinic or as a consult, inpatient, or outpatient attending. Illustrate points with short vignettes with memorable x-ray, pathology, colonoscopy, or surgical findings. This is a wonderful way to enhance learner interest in and retention of your major points. Alternatively, have learners work through cases in small or large groups to discuss key elements pertaining to your objectives.

Are you required to hand in a syllabus for your presentation or to create a handout? Check and recheck the desired format of the syllabus. What is the due date? What is the required length and word count? How should the references be listed? Should all authors be listed or just the first three? Ask for an example of a prior syllabus that the course directors think is good and could act as your guide.

Your audience hopes for a focused, clear, and logical presentation. Straightforward, transparent objectives help, as does a logical progression (Hatton 1982; Whitman and Schwenk 1997). To make your presentation logical, begin by talking out loud; this will help identify the non sequiturs, fuzzy thinking, out-of-place data, illogical order of facts, or overabundance of visual material for the time slot. It is never too early to begin speaking your main points aloud. I do this because it enables me to hear inconsistencies or hesitancies and any inability to smoothly explain content and concepts. Missing segues and links become obvious. How are you getting from point A to point B? Missing pieces of information surface when you start speaking. The excessive use of *you know* and *like* becomes readily apparent as you listen to yourself explain a concept to a mirror. The mirror will not answer you back as it did in the Walt Disney movie *Snow White,* but it will be an asset to you in your quest to sound polished and to look upbeat, confident, knowledgeable, and relaxed.

Exploration involves using multiple types of question to understand your material during your preparation phase. Exploration is fun, engaging, and enlightening. The exploration step is perfect for preparing for a small-group discussion, but what does it have to do with preparing for a lecture, attending rounds, or conducting a physical diagnosis session? Exploration means obtaining the evidence and critically reviewing it before presenting it as fact. Exploring with your own questions permits you to successfully anticipate your audience's questions, concerns, and points of confusion. It also helps you to create an order that makes sense. Frequently, the exploration phase occurs when the teacher recognizes that some or all of the learners will be missing a link, bridge, or segues to understanding the material. Once your knowledge base is clear, use questions to dissect it and make it relevant to your teaching goals.

At the time of your presentation, use questions to smoothly manage the group dynamics and create the right atmosphere for learning. Consider asking questions and answering them yourself during your presentation to maximize the learning. Multiple types of question are useful. Table 4.2 shows a partial list of the types of question.

Table 4.2. Types of Question

Open ended: "What's going on?"

Informational: "What is meant by portal hypertension?"

Diagnostic: "What test might help you determine this?"

Extension: "How would you proceed after obtaining this result?"

Challenge: "Why do you say that?"

Priority: "Of the three tests, which would you order first, and why?"

Action: "What would you do next?"

Prediction: "Given the lab values, what do you predict her biopsy will show?"

Summarizing and generalizing: "How would you summarize this case?" "How would you apply the lessons learned to another case?"

Source: Adapted from Louis Barnes, PhD, and James Honan, EdD, Harvard Graduate School of Education, Developing Discussion Leadership Skills Course, 2003.

Step 3. Presentation

Don't let yourself down with weak presentation skills after all the effort you have spent researching the topic. Most lecture presentations begin with optimism and excitement, but then meander and lose their sizzle in the middle, coming back at the end to hammer home a few points. The audience waits for the end, with its potential enlightenment and encapsulated summary of what was discussed. Small groups also begin with high expectations but can quickly degenerate into gabfests or silent standoffs unless you, as the leader, are skillfully prepared to help the group maneuver through the essential material and encourage discussion of the objectives in a lively give-and-take manner. Laboratory exercises may not reach the objectives set forth in the syllabus or guide for the laboratory unless the laboratory leader is facile, knowledgeable, organized, and goal oriented.

Practice

The best way to ensure success in the presentation step is to make an outline of your talk, discussion questions, laboratory cases, or workshop activities. The outline can be sketchy at this point because it will change, but make sure you have a basic roadmap. This roadmap should include each visual and each word slide. The outline will help you organize the logical order of your visuals, questions and cases, data, transitions, and summary slides.

Begin to talk out loud early on, starting with your introduction, then moving into the body of your presentation, followed by your summary points. You will quickly see if the logic and length is off the mark. Limit the number of visuals to essential slides. The biggest teaching error I see at grand rounds or continuing medical education talks is too many slides for the time allotted. Each slide generally requires one to three minutes to discuss.

For small or large groups, sketch out several different types of question to ask.

Practice being enthusiastic. You have done intensive preparation and explored your material from all angles; now you need to present your work in an enthusiastic and knowledgeable manner. Enthusiasm is a cultivated asset of excellent teachers. It wins you brownie points and accolades as long as it is accompanied by real knowledge and a thoughtful, logical approach. Don't wait to have an enthusiastic tone of voice until the day of your presentation. You may be too nervous then. Memorize your enthusiasm.

Practice presenting in an upbeat but unhurried pace that allows you to cover your material in the allotted time. Extensive behind-the-scenes practice is generally needed to distill the mountain of material into a few memorable points.

Fast forward in your mind to the hotel or conference center with an auditorium full of people or a small conference room full of eager learners, all of whom have paid money and are taking precious free time to hear expert lectures for continuing medical education credit. Did you practice sufficiently to make the material your own? Did you send your slide set ahead to the audiovisual assistant? Anticipate disaster so that, no matter what happens, you can carry on.

Practice using at least one to three minutes as the time allotment for each slide. If your talk is twenty minutes, you should have no more than fifteen slides. Otherwise, you will be rushing rather than adequately talking about each of them. No one slide is indispensable. Walk through your presentation; find slides you can say instead of show.

If you are a discussion leader, prepare more questions than you will have time for. While some questions could lead to ten to twenty minutes of discussion, others could lead to blank stares or uncomfortable shifting in seats. Because each discussion group is different, it is hard to estimate the number of questions needed to adequately cover the material. Have questions in reserve.

As a laboratory leader, you will be expected to cover the cases, slides, movies, and microscope exercises smoothly and effectively. Know your material and be prepared to lead even when students are only moderately interested. Using questions, audience-response systems, or team-based learning will make the group more active in the learning process.

For workshops, leaders need to estimate the time for activities carefully to give participants enough time to do the planned exercises and go over them as a group, so as to hear the differences and similarities.

Build reiteration and review of crucial points into your teaching exercises. Reiteration of important points will help to solidify the concepts to take home. Find ways of saying the same thing differently. Show the concept from new angles. Use visual aids, diagrams, and photographs to emphasize and solidify your learners' understanding.

Clarify and simplify your talk. It will pay off with excellent evaluations.

Delivery

If you have prepared, by the time the presentation comes, you will welcome the opportunity to give your polished teaching session. If you have not prepared, presentation day will be unpleasant.

To stop the jitters the day of your delivery, put your mind on pleasing thoughts. I think of my husband and son smiling at me and being proud that I did a good job. I know how unhappy their expressions will be if I tell them at dinner that the talk was a disaster because I panicked, could not work the LCD projector, forgot my memory stick, or was unable to show the slides for a technical reason. I do well so that I can celebrate afterward. I make sure that I give the presentation my best shot. I wish to move on to whatever deadline is waiting in the wings, not in defeat but in victory. Another way I diminish anxiety is to put the focus on having the group enjoy learning from me. My heart-pounding diminishes as I see that the learner seems to be learning and enjoying it.

On the day before and the day of your presentation, eat and drink carefully. Eat what makes you comfortable and fortified. I shop or buy extra comfort food so that I have enough for the day of teaching. Comfort food for me is chicken and rice. For someone else it may be bread, potatoes, vegetables, ground meat, tofu, or crackers and cheese. Avoid gassy foods. Avoid foods that promote extra bowel movements. You do not wish to be in the bathroom longer than necessary when you have last-minute things to do.

Be careful of celebratory dinners the night before. Celebrating to excess with alcoholic drinks and going to bed late the night before a big presentation, lecture, workshop, or discussion group is not a good idea. Your wits need to be as sharp as possible. You can celebrate after your lectures are finished.

Find out where you will get coffee. Will you make it in your room or are you at a hotel where you need to order it? Should you get your coffee the night before and reheat it so you don't have to wait in line?

Get up early to practice at least one more time. On the morning of the presentation, I memorize segues so that my presentation flows smoothly. Set the alarm or have the hotel operator wake you up so that you do not miss this all-important last-minute practice. I set the alarm early enough to have time to go through my talk at least once and preferably twice. This may mean that I am waking up at 4 a.m. Final practices ensure that I know my talk well, including my introductory comments and transitions.

Lay out your clothes the night before or put everything in one spot in your closet, including belt, tie, scarf, pocketbook, shoes. You may realize that your silver pin is tarnished, your shoes scuffed, your tie has a grease spot and you need to pick another, or your skirt has a stain in the front. Before being a first-time moderator of a scientific session at a national meeting, I spent so much time making up questions to ask each oral presenter that I never took the time to put on the outfit I had brought for the occasion. Instead, I wore a casual outfit that was out of step with being a moderator. Look the part! Your audience expects you to look your best. Cameras may flash during and at the end of your presentation. Focus on looking polished and professional.

Arrive at your meeting place at least thirty minutes early. Thirty minutes is the minimum time I would leave for setup; I prefer forty-five to sixty minutes. This prepresentation time always goes quickly as you note the missing pointer, awkward podium, absent flip chart, nonfunctioning LCD projector, nonexistent extension cord or power strip, and no new battery for the slide advancer.

Know the podium area. Go over the lights, LCD projector, and microphone, raising and lowering the screen. Check the laser pointer and have a backup laser pointer, and know how to use both. Consider bringing a traditional pointer that collapses. If you will use the blackboard, make sure it is clean. Have a backup presentation on a memory stick. I bring a 3 x 5 inch index card with final reminders and transition phrases I worry that I will forget. I place this on the podium with my watch, a bottle or glass of water, and a tissue, in case I sneeze.

If there are steps to the podium, test them, to be sure you do not fall or lurch to your talk. Steps may be uneven, too high, or too low. They can have lips or tread that is easy to trip on if you are wearing high heels. Go up and down the stairs so that you know them and will not fall in the darkened conference room.

Make a connection to your audience by smiling at early arrivals and introducing yourself to them. Break the ice for yourself by interacting in a kind and pleasant manner before your presentation.

When the time comes for you to be introduced by the moderator, make sure to smile and look pleasant. This will give you an immediate bond to your learners and help each of them feel more enthusiastic about learning from you.

Don't spend your time standing behind the podium, but get out from behind it to tell a disarming story, anecdote, or clinical vignette. Standing in front or to the side of it enables you to be seen. Don't be afraid to move around. Make sure your microphone, if it has a cord, permits you to move. Ask for a cordless microphone in the setup time before your presentation. If you are early enough, the audiovisual person may find one for you, unchaining you from the podium. If there is no remote slide advancer, you need to advance your slides or ask someone else to do it.

You will never be too early to set up for a presentation, but being even a bit late will rob you of valuable moments to organize your thoughts, note the treacherous steps, the glaring lights in your face, the missing remote, the lack of sufficient chairs for your small group, the heavily scribbled-on blackboard that you may need to clean off, the remnant lunches, bottles, or garbage that has to be thrown away in your small-group room to create a welcoming space. These disconcerting features of your presentation space can be improved if you arrive early, but they are immutable negatives if you run in late and cannot fix them.

Scan the audience or group for friendly or interested faces. The whole room desires your gaze. Make sure that you turn your gaze to both sides of the room.

Remember to have at your place or on the podium a pen and pad or 3 x 5 inch cards to make notes and take down questions.

Speak with the audiovisual person if one is assigned to you or your room. The personal connection you have established helps when things start to go wrong. Go over the use or nonuse of the podium buttons. What are you responsible for doing? What will the audiovisual person do, and what are you expected to do? How do you do it? What happens if an error occurs?

Have a clock, watch, or timer present to help you keep stay within your time limit. It is important to start and end on time. Starting late angers the early arrivals and ending late angers both the audience and all who come after you. It is your job to have practiced sufficiently to know that your presentation will end on time.

Let your presentation be smooth and free of jarring notes. Look prepared. Memorize your talk so that if your slides fail or you lose your notes or list of questions, you will be able to give your presentation anyway.

Summary with Schematic

Don't be surprised if some members of your audience seem to perk up when you begin your summary. A short (two- to five-minute) summary with a diagram of the major concepts or points is an excellent way to have learners "take away" the knowledge and build on it by their own reading and studying. Carefully consider, in your preparation phase, what your key points are. Do not give a complete relisting of your talk; rather, specifically pick out a few points that are key. Leave the rest off the list for simplicity. The summary is your opportunity to clarify, emphasize, and distill. It is your final chance to hammer home your major message. Make that message succinct. Use a visual aid, if appropriate, to emphasize your bottom line.

Step 4. Realizations and Reflection

I both love and hate the realizations-and-reflection step because it forces me to honestly review my teaching for better or for worse. I push myself to reflect immediately, again the following day, and once more at a later date. I write down my ideas for change, as well as what went well.

Recently, I gave grand rounds on colon cancer screening with another speaker. The presentation could not start because the electric cord to the LCD projector did not reach the outlet in the conference room. It took about ten minutes to locate an extension cord with power strip. The combination laser pointer and slide advancer stopped working after about five minutes, and no battery was available to fix it. A volunteer from the audience had to be recruited to advance the slides. These problems could have been anticipated. I made mental notes to bring a pointer and AA battery of my own and pack an extension cord/power strip in my briefcase. Extra equipment is worthwhile, especially at a previously unknown location. Alternatively, call ahead and ask to have a power strip and AA batteries ready.

The day after a presentation or workshop is generally the best time to consider changes to improve. You should have access to paper or computer-based evaluations of your performance. You will have a chance to review, at least tentatively, if you succeeded or failed. Congratulatory messages may come in. Carefully read each evaluation for helpful comments. Try not to be too disturbed if hurtful comments as well as helpful comments are written. I say hurtful, because over the years as a course director, I have seen examples of unpleasant, unkind, and downright rude comments about teachers from students, learners, and colleagues.

Teachers worry too much or too little about their evaluations. Recently, I gave a talk that I thought was good and I received nice compliments and applause at the end. The evaluations were significantly less than stellar. It took me hours to stop rehashing the evaluations in my mind. What was wrong? Eventually, I recognized from rereading the comments that I had failed to pitch the talk at the right level. It was an excellent talk, just not for the training level that I had been asked to address. I had thought a lot about the talk, but I had spent little time putting myself at the level of the audience and asking what the objectives should be for these learners. The learners were clear in their evaluations. The lecture was off the mark because it was pitched at a higher level of training. I had not addressed the needs of the learners. Rather, I had given the talk that I wished to give and enjoyed giving. Thus, the less-than-ideal evaluations I received.

Step 5. Refinement

After each teaching exercise's evaluations have come in, I go over the changes I would like to make for the next time. For the pathophysiology course I direct, we invite all students to a feedback session where all comments, positive and negative, can be aired. The course administrator serves as the note taker. Afterward, I review each comment with the course manager, forming a list to use for changing the next year's course. I also sit down with my teaching fellow and course manager and ask each of them to provide suggestions for change from what they have noted and from their reading of the anonymous student evaluations, sent in several weeks after the end of the course. Together, we make a list of suggested changes. Then I call a meeting of the advisory committee for the course and ask the committee members for their opinion on the changes we are contemplating. I weigh each suggestion for its ability to move the course to a better level of teaching. The committee drops a few suggestions after discussion; others form the basis for the major work to be done for the next year. Minor changes or complaints noted during the course are rectified immediately.

View Negative Evaluations as Opportunities for Improvement

A common realizations-and-reflection mistake is to focus anger on the negative evaluations and evaluators. No matter how hurtful, there is often a kernel of truth in the negative evaluations, just as there is truth in the positives. The positive evaluations count just as much as, if not more than, the negatives, though it rarely seems that way when the negative evaluations roll in and take immediate prominence in your thinking about what you spent a large chunk of time preparing. Before I read every evaluation, I think to myself, how would I have rated this teaching session if I were the learner? Knowing what I think were the strengths and weaknesses of my own teaching, or those of someone teaching in a course that I direct, enables me to be more dispassionate about both the criticisms and the praise as I read the evaluations. I understand why something negative is being said because I saw the same problem but hoped others would not. As you go over the evaluations, make notes that can be entered into a permanent log, book, or Web site. What is wrong will be fixed; what is right will be perpetuated. After reading all the evaluations and noting the numerical grades, list your top choices for change. I do not slavishly follow each and every suggestion for change, but most of my awards for teaching were won because I made changes based on negative reviews. The ability to change in response to criticism is what distinguishes successful teachers from unsuccessful teachers.

Guaranteed Methods of Engaging Your Audience

Put yourself in the audience's shoes and you will soon recognize what makes learners happy: discovering new knowledge, exploring ideas and concepts, actively participating, being recognized, heard, and respected. Giving them something to think about, to do, and to create (Allen and Tanner 2005; Knight and Wood 2005) is a foolproof way of engaging the audience.

How do you do this? Ask questions of your audience even in the large forum of grand rounds; organize breakout groups to create a new method for doing something or to understand a difficult medical concept or new procedure. Use small buzz groups to get people to talk to each other about a specific question or problem that you clearly pose. After ten to fifteen minutes, have groups present their findings and a summary. Ask one learner to explain what he or she understands about a topic to another learner or to the whole group. Use an audience-response system (Wood 2004) or team-based learning (Michaelsen and Sweet 2008b) to assure engagement. Everyone benefits from and enjoys being a part of an actively learning group.

Common Mistakes and How to Avoid Them

The most common mistake in teaching is having too much content in the lecture or small-group session for the time allotted. Other mistakes are not anticipating problems before they occur, such as not having sent your slide presentation beforehand to the administrator responsible for hosting your grand rounds or invited presentation, not arriving early enough to open and check your presentation for accuracy, not having a backup slide presentation on a memory stick, or not having an LCD projector that works. These errors can simply be avoided by visualizing your presentation and the consequences of your slides not being available for your lecture and taking practical steps to avoid this disaster.

Other common mistakes are having slides populated with numbers that are not going to be easily visible or readily grasped, and reading directly from slides with no annotation to help the audience grasp your perspective. Apologizing for dense or incomprehensible slides is common. When I hear those apologies, I wonder why the speaker did not take the time to delete the slide instead of apologizing for it. If you need to apologize, get rid of the offending object. It frequently seems as if the lecturer has not looked at his or her presentation since the last time of giving the talk and has forgotten to remove the too densely numbered slide. Slide mistakes fall under errors in preparation. Have someone with a good eye view your slide show critically and honestly tell you which slides are essential and which slides can be skipped because you can say what is on them without the visual aids. Each slide takes from one to three minutes to present. If you have forty-five minutes, the number of slides you can safely show is in the range of thirty or fewer.

Not starting on time when some but not all of the audience is there is a mistake in the presentation category. Begin at the time listed for your presentation, or at the most five minutes later. Do not wait for a quorum. If you feel uncomfortable starting your presentation before more people arrive, engage the audience by asking them questions about themselves. Remember how uncomfortable you will be when you do not have time to complete your slide set or people walk out before you finish because you started late. People who arrived on time are going to downgrade your teaching ability when you hold them hostage to your wanting more people to be present before starting. This attitude is a slap in the face to those who arrived on time. These people should be rewarded, not punished.

Mistakes in summarizing generally take the form of excessive length. Stay within five minutes and it is truly a summary; more time and you are recreating your talk.

Examples of What Can and Does Go Wrong

Three recent teaching assignments did not go as well as they might have, largely because I failed to follow my own framework for success. I will walk you through each assignment to show where I went wrong and what I would do differently the next time.

In the first assignment, I was asked to be the expert consultant at an internal medicine weekly conference for house staff regarding an elevated alkaline phosphatase to greater than 1000 IU/dL in a patient with an osteomyelitis of the foot. The gamma glutamyl transpeptidase was greater than 500 IU, indicating that the alkaline phosphatase was of liver rather than bone origin. My job was to explain what I thought caused the elevation and why.

What steps did I complete? I completed my preparation step by doing a thorough job of researching the topic, including classic articles and recent articles on alkaline phosphatase elevation in patients without intrinsic liver disease, but with other illnesses, such as Hodgkin disease, congestive heart failure, or sepsis. I synthesized the information in my head and was very enthusiastic about all that I had learned. I had spent lots of time in preparation and none in visualization. I never bothered to take even one or two minutes to imagine how I was going to transmit the information I had so carefully gleaned to a small audience of tired residents, interns, and students on a Friday morning. I had information in my head but no clear plan of how to deliver it. I also never wrote out my objectives or said them out loud. Writing down or saying my objectives for the elevated alkaline phosphatase enzyme picture would have taken only a minute. Then, I would have been able to visualize an orderly and logical progression of information and concepts, building up to a conclusion with a tidy and powerful summary. In addition to not visualizing or defining my objectives, I did not maximize interaction with the audience in the presentation step. I failed to use my favorite tool of questions to engage an audience. I did not ask the audience questions about their differential before I gave my "expert" opinion. Questions that ask the audience to think and work to solve the patient's complex problem are a sure-fire method for engaging the entire room. I lectured at the audience rather than engaging them in a give-and-take discussion. The take-home points are (1) visualize your performance from the beginning, (2) write down objectives even for a ten-minute presentation, (3) have a plan for engaging your audience with questions to show their understanding of the problem, (4) summarize at the end, and (5) use a visual method for explaining concepts, even if it is a flip chart or white board with marker pens.

Assignment 2 was for a continuing medical education course on cancer diagnosis and treatment for primary care physicians. I was asked to moderate a three-person panel on colon cancer. The panel was to focus on failure to diagnose or follow-up on rectal bleeding. We had a thirty-five-minute time slot. Each panelist was asked to speak for eight minutes. This plan left about ten minutes for a question-and-answer period. I had been panel moderator for this same topic the previous year. Our talk had run over into the subsequent lecturer's time and we'd had no time for questions. I resolved not to have our talks run over again. Each of us agreed to cut our time allotment to eight minutes by cutting the number of slides we showed. The day before the panel discussion, I sent out an e-mail reminding each panelist to practice so that ten minutes could be left for questions. What happened? The three panelists, including me, finished the presentations leaving only two minutes for discussion. I took two questions from the floor, but many hands were raised to ask other questions that I did not address. I announced that the panelists would be available during the coffee break ninety minutes later to answer questions. The disgruntled audience did ask questions during the break time, but this was clearly less than optimal because excellent questions were asked, which all participants should have heard along with the answers to them. What steps did I fail? I failed the visualization and presentation steps. I never imagined myself doing a direct intervention, for example, standing up behind a co-panelist if he or she ran over. When a panelist did begin to run overtime, I did not activate what should have been a prearranged signaling system to indicate the need for him or her to go to the last slide and finish abruptly. As a result, we lost our panel's question period two years in a row and gained the ill will of an eager and sophisticated audience with numerous questions.

In assignment 3, I gave a lecture during the annual Abdominal Exam session for second-year Harvard Medical School students entitled "Why is it difficult to diagnose the origin of abdominal pain?" I had given this talk many times before, and it had been well received. However, the amount of time for the talk was cut from twenty minutes to twelve. I ignored this cut in time and plowed ahead with the same number of slides—fifteen, an excessive number for a twelve-minute talk. I failed on the presentation step because I did not take the time to weed out nonessential slides and rework the talk. Not surprisingly, my overall score fell, and I received a number of student comments saying that I spoke too fast and presented too much material in the time interval. This was not unexpected, but the comments hurt. I will cut the number of slides for next year's talk, and it will be a better learning experience for the audience.

In summary, a framework provides an essential tool for a medical teacher to give memorable and active learning sessions. Visualization with the creation of transparent objectives, intensive preparation with questions to guide the exploration of the material, a polished presentation with clear distillation of concepts and a summary, the realization of how you did through your own and others' evaluations, and reflection leading to change—together these steps ensure success.

✒ TEACHING TIPS

1. Caring deeply about your learners' learning is an important quality to nurture.
2. Follow a framework for approaching each new assignment.
3. Start with imagining how you will do the assignment, and specify what you hope your learners will learn from you (objectives).
4. Say your objectives out loud.
5. Prepare intensively, even if you have given the talk before.
6. Be current and evidence-based with your literature review.
7. Beware of cramming too much content into too short a time frame.
8. Practice in front of a mirror and assess your expressions; listen to your tone of voice. Is it upbeat, confident, and energetic? If not, work on making it so.
9. Reiterate and review during your presentation; make it seem like fun by using images, diagrams, and case material.
10. Summarize succinctly. Consider using a diagram to convey concepts.

✄ TAKE-HOME POINTS

- Anticipate all possible problems; they will all occur at one time or another.
- Visualize yourself being successful and getting applause; this vision will drive you to prepare properly.
- Arrive early enough to catch set-up mistakes and audiovisual glitches and to get comfortable with your surroundings.
- Be enthusiastic; enthusiasm is contagious.
- Pay close attention to your evaluations. Do not toss them out. Find out what was liked, and why; try to duplicate this.
- Teacher evaluations do not lie; they need to be understood if you are to improve and stay on top.
- Take your learners seriously; they are your customers/clients in the competitive world of medical teaching.

CHAPTER FIVE

Understanding Adult Learning Theory, Bloom's Taxonomy of Objectives, Critical Thinking, and Curriculum Development

- *What are the major principles of adult learning?*
- *What is Bloom's Taxonomy of Objectives?*
- *What does critical thinking mean?*
- *What is the "six-step approach" to curriculum development?*
- *How do I get the new curriculum off the ground?*

Understanding Educational Terms

The words *adult learning theory* may strike terror into your heart when you first hear them. However, knowledge of adult learning theory translates into practical principles that are valuable to know before teaching adults. Bloom's Taxonomy of Objectives sounds like a stuffed bird rather than a desirable educational tool, while "critical thinking" leaves you guessing at what is meant and wishing you were in the "insiders" club of educators who understand these terms. *Curriculum,* the official name for what you are planning to teach, depends for its success on your understanding some important aspects of adult learning theory, objectives, and critical thinking. I will briefly explain each term and show its utility for you as the developer of new curriculum.

Adult Learning Theory

If *pedagogy* refers to the art and science of educating children through a teacher-focused approach, *andragogy* refers to the art and science of helping adults learn through a learner-focused rather than a teacher-focused educational process. Learning is defined as the acquisition of knowledge, habits, attitudes, or behavior and involves change. David Kolb (1984, 38) notes that "learning is the process whereby knowledge is created through the transformation of experience." Teacher-focused education is the way children learn, with the teacher designing, leading the exercise, and directing what is to be learned. Malcolm Knowles (1990), a respected college educator, used the term *andragogy* to separate adult's learning needs from children's learning needs. Adults want to understand what and why they are learning, and they want to be involved in creating educational activities. Adults' prior and present life experiences count and modify their learning.

Professor Knowles focused on the following characteristics of adult learners:

- Adults want to know why they are expected to learn something.
- Adults' life experiences color their learning.
- Adults approach learning as a problem-solving exercise.
- Adults appreciate immediate applicability.

Medical students, residents, fellows, faculty members, and participants in continuing medical education exercises are all adult learners.

Application to Curriculum Development

What do these characteristics tell us about the types of educational exercise to select for adults? The following types of exercise are useful, particularly in a small-group format, for engaging the adult learner.

1. Case-based learning
2. Role-playing exercises
3. Simulations
4. Self-evaluation exercises
5. Team-based learning
6. Audience-response systems

Adults enjoy and learn best from active learning, in which participants work in small groups on a real project or problem (Galbraith 1998; Knowles, Holton, and Swanson 2005). Diverse adult groups include members with expert knowledge and those with various life experiences. This allows each member to contribute significantly. Group members benefit from teaching coaches who act as organizers, facilitators, and overall motivators. Small-group activities provide the opportunity to share, reflect, and generalize the learning experiences.

Adults want to be involved in the planning and evaluation of their learning. Life experiences, including errors, provide an important basis for some of the learning activities. Adults, because they are goal oriented, are most interested in learning subjects that have immediate relevance to their job or personal life. Adult learning is oriented to problem solving rather than mastering content.

Bloom's Taxonomy of Objectives

Objectives are the teacher's way of communicating what he or she wants students to learn. Objectives should be well thought out. Bloom's Taxonomy of Objectives (Bloom et al. 1956) refers to a framework for classifying categories of objectives along a continuum of increasingly complex levels of learning. Objectives help students attain these higher levels of learning. Bloom's classification is helpful in a practical sense because your learning exercises, lectures, and small-group activities should all be aligned with the objectives you have decided on.

Definition of an Objective

An objective contains a noun and a verb. The verb describes the type of thought process that you wish the students to attain, while the noun explains the knowledge that you wish the students to learn. Objectives are what you want the end result of the learning process to be and are simply tools to help teachers communicate and make clear to one another and to the students what the student is expected to learn (Anderson and Krathwohl 2001; Marzano and Kendall 2007).

In his classic treatise, Bloom outlined six sequential stages of increasingly complex cognitive thinking:

1. Knowledge
2. Comprehension
3. Application
4. Analysis
5. Synthesis
6. Evaluation

Definitions of Terms

Knowledge is information retrieval and is considered the lowest level of thought process.

Comprehension, the next level of thinking, means learning new knowledge after a verbal or nonverbal communication. The three ways for demonstrating comprehension in the taxonomy are translation, interpretation, and extrapolation. *Translation* means encoding information received into a different form, *interpretation* means reworking ideas into a new configuration, and *extrapolation* means making inferences and predictions from the information received.

Application is the third level of cognition and refers to abstractions being correctly used in a new problem without the student's being prompted.

Analysis is the recognition of relationships between parts of knowledge and the way they are organized.

Synthesis means creating new knowledge from what has been given.

Evaluation means deciding on the value of the knowledge learned.

Lessons begin with objectives containing a verb and a noun, for example, "List four causes of chest pain." These drive the instruction and curriculum design. The teaching exercises must be designed to achieve the objectives. Objectives can and should bring in multiple cognitive levels. Assessment of teaching exercises focuses on whether the objectives have been achieved.

Creating Objectives for Preclinical and Clinical Teaching

Stuart and Krauser (2000) note that drawing up objectives helps students learn and makes evaluation of their performance easier. Objectives, according to these authors, should be

SMART:
S specific
M measurable
A attainable
R relevant
T time-framed

Objectives are what you hope the student, resident, or peer group will learn and take away from your program, presentation, course, or workshop. A *specific* objective refers to what you want the learner to be able to do or know— what, how, when, and under what circumstances. Stuart and Krauser (2000) note that it is imperative that the objective be *measurable* or assessable so that the learner can demonstrate, list, describe, explain, or discuss it. Skills can be measured for how well they are performed and how long it takes to do them. *Attainable* signifies that the objective is a reasonable expectation given the educational program. Objectives should be *relevant* to the goal of the educational activity and *time-framed*, or "achievable by the end."

Examples of objectives include:

Preclinical tutorial on pathophysiology of small and large bowel diseases:
1. Name the common pathogens that cause food poisoning and state the timing of onset of diarrhea after ingesting the tainted food.
2. Define diarrhea. Discuss secretory diarrhea and compare and contrast it to osmotic diarrhea, diarrhea secondary to exudative diseases, and diarrhea secondary to motility disorders of the intestine.

Preclinical introduction to the abdominal examination for second-year students:
1. Using your knowledge of innervation and embryology, explain why it is difficult to diagnose the origin of abdominal pain.
2. Demonstrate the physical diagnosis maneuvers to exclude the presence of an enlarged spleen tip.

Clinical skills for medical students and residents:
1. List five characteristics of abdominal pain that should be asked about in taking the history from any patient with abdominal pain.
2. Describe or demonstrate the best way to examine the ticklish patient's abdomen.

Faculty development for small group discussion leadership:
1. Name four types of question that are helpful to use in small-group learning.
2. Explain two methods for increasing the quiet student's contributions in a small-group discussion class and two methods for decreasing the dominant student's contributions to the class.

Postgraduate learning:
1. Describe the effects of obesity on the lower esophageal sphincter and the possible relationship to the recognized increase in adenocarcinoma of the distal esophagus.
2. Outline the local and systemic mechanisms that lead to nonsteroidal anti-inflammatory drug damage of the gastric mucosa.

Critical Thinking

Ennis (1962, 83) used the definition of "critical thinking" as the "correct assessing of statements." In his classic article, "A Concept of Critical Thinking," Ennis listed twelve aspects of critical thinking. In addition to (1) grasping the meaning of a statement, one must judge whether:

2. there is ambiguity in a line of reasoning
3. certain statements contradict each other
4. a conclusion follows necessarily
5. a statement is specific enough
6. a statement is the application of a certain principle
7. an observation statement is reliable
8. an inductive conclusion is warranted
9. the problem has been identified
10. something is an assumption
11. a definition is adequate
12. a statement made by an alleged authority is acceptable

Later, Ennis (1985, 45) provided a broader definition: "Critical thinking is reflective and reasonable thinking that is focused on deciding what to believe or do." He noted that creative activities covered by this definition include formulating hypotheses, asking questions, devising alternatives, and making plans for experiments. He emphasized that critical thinking is a practical activity because deciding what to believe or do is of practical value. If the concept of critical thinking is compared to "higher-order thinking" skills and Bloom's taxonomy's top three levels of classifying educational objectives, namely, analysis, synthesis, and evaluation, Ennis believes that critical thinking is the "directly practical side of higher-order thinking," given that it is focused on deciding what to believe or what to do.

A critical thinker has the following attitude and disposition:

- Is open minded
- Is fair minded
- Searches for evidence
- Asks questions
- Tries to be well informed
- Is attentive to others' views and reasons
- Has beliefs that reflect the best available evidence
- Is willing to consider alternatives and revise beliefs

Ennis (1985) described four sets of abilities that are constitutive of critical thinking: (1) abilities related to clarity, (2) abilities related to establishing a sound knowledge base for inference, (3) abilities related to inference (i.e., deduction, induction, value judging), and (4) abilities involved in going about decision making in an orderly and useful way, that is, problem solving. The critical thinker should be clear in the problem-solving process about what is going on. While solving problems, the critical thinker is interacting with others to make decisions about beliefs or actions. Ennis says that critical thinking can be taught.

A critical thinking process has these components:

- Identifying and analyzing the problem
- Clarifying meanings
- Gathering the evidence
- Assessing the evidence
- Inferring conclusions
- Making an overall judgment

In the future, the national board examinations will pay more attention to critical thinking skills and problem-solving skills. The National Board will ask students and residents to demonstrate data- and information-gathering skills, as well as to analyze, evaluate, and assess scientific, clinical, and pharmacologic data presented to them in problem-solving exercises.

Critical thinking is useful in all branches of medicine, from clinical practice to research and education. Training physicians to think critically by learning to ask questions, solve problems, gather and assess evidence, and draw conclusions is an essential but complicated process (Jenicek and Hitchcock 2005). The curriculum should be designed as an opportunity to showcase these components of critical thinking.

Doctors are expected to be critical thinkers. Creating a curriculum with opportunities for modeling the important and learned attributes of questioning, problem solving, data gathering, and evaluating and assessing evidence should be promoted.

What Is a Curriculum?

Curriculum is defined as a planned instructional experience designed to give learners specific knowledge and skills (Kern, Thomas, and Hughes 2009). The word comes from the Latin word *currere,* for a racecourse that needs to be run around or covered. Hill (2007) notes that curricula should be continuously revised for what we teach and how we teach it because of changes in culture, teaching technologies, teaching staff, stakeholder interests, and resources. Kern, Thomas, and Hughes developed a logical and methodical approach to creating new curricula for medical education. Their 2009 book outlines a six-step approach.

Step 1. The Problem to Solve

Before creating new educational material, determine what you want to teach and why. Identify a deficiency or gap in learning, and this becomes the problem you wish to solve. What do the learners ideally need to know in contrast to what is currently being taught? Do they need to know this material for an examination, the national boards, clinics, attending rounds, licensure examinations, or just for good medical care? A general-needs assessment refers to the difference between the current and the ideal approaches to educating learners on a specific topic (Bass 2009). The ideal approach includes "identifying the appropriate target audience, the appropriate content, the best educational strategies and the best evaluation methods" (15). A task analysis focuses on the specific list of tasks that needs to be accomplished to solve the problem. Generally, the first task is learning the literature. Next, expert opinions help in the design; design groups and telephone interviews of experts are useful. If you are starting a completely new curriculum, you will likely spend a great deal of time weighing and deciding what needs to be taught.

Step 2. Learners' Needs

You need to know what the learners already know or are being taught in order to decide what the gaps in their curriculum are. Ask the learners their perceptions of what is missing. Look at evaluations of the prior year's course and jot down the complaints of what was not taught well, or not at all. Ask your teachers what their top three subjects are that need to be added, revamped, or dropped. Hold informal or formal interviews or focus groups with students, residents, fellows, and faculty to pinpoint deficiencies. Send out questionnaires with unambiguous questions; use direct observations, tests, audits of current performance, and strategic planning sessions to identify what should be the basis for your new curriculum effort.

Step 3. Goals and Objectives

Goals and objectives are the ends toward which the teaching effort is addressed (Thomas 2009). They should be carefully written and be unambiguous. Thomas defines a *goal* as a broad educational objective, while *objective* refers to specific measurable knowledge, behaviors, attitudes, or skills. Objectives should provide the "game plan" for the educational exercise. Goals and objectives tell those involved as teachers or learners what the curriculum is designed to do.

The basic elements for objectives are:

1. Who
2. Will do
3. How well or how much
4. Of what
5. By when

Write the objectives without ambiguity. They should clearly convey what is wanted. Objectives can refer to different levels of learning, as Bloom pointed out. Thus, learners may be responsible for increasing their knowledge, changing an attitude, or practicing a skill. Each objective is written to enable teachers and learners to strive to complete the desired curriculum. Ask an outsider to read the goals and objectives to see if they are unambiguous. It is important to have a reasonable but not an excessive number of objectives; you want to provide direction for the curriculum but do not want to dampen creativity and curiosity.

Step 4. Educational Strategies

Teachers align the objectives with the teaching methods. The amount of time, faculty, facilities, money, and clinical material need to be factored into the method chosen. Strategies will include both content—what is to be taught—and methods—the ways in which the content can be presented. The course planner needs to link the objectives with the teaching methods chosen. Thus, if you choose a cognitive or knowledge objective, then a lecture or facilitated discussion may be best, whereas for an affective or attitudinal objective, real-life experiences coupled with a group discussion may be more useful than a lecture, while psychomotor or skill objectives may best be accomplished in a simulation laboratory, or the demonstration of the skill may be videotaped for review by learners and faculty.

Writing objectives is a learned skill. Use verbs that are "open to few interpretations" (Thomas 2009, 44), such as *list, define, describe,* followed by what you will specifically cover.

Methods for accomplishing objectives vary. Table 5.1 summarizes the various objectives and the common methods for achieving them.

Table 5.1.   Objectives, and Methods for Achieving Them

Cognitive: knowledge or problem solving
  Readings
  Lectures
  Audiovisual aids
  Discussion
  Programmed learning

Affective: attitudinal
  Discussion groups
  Clinical interactions

Psychomotor skills: behavioral or performance skill
  Procedural skills in out-patient clinics and in-patient areas
  Simulation laboratories
  Video reviews

Source: Adapted from Thomas 2009.

Step 5. Implementation

Starting a new curriculum generally requires people and money. You need to identify what resources are necessary to get the curriculum off the ground and headed in the right direction. Who will help? How will they be paid? What is the time frame? Where will the teaching exercises be held? Who will do the assessment? How much will it cost?

Step 6. Evaluation and Feedback

How did the new curriculum go? Think through how the curriculum will be evaluated before the new curriculum is launched. Evaluation and feedback set the stage for improvement for the next time. Faculty members will gain insight into what might have been done better, while learners will see how much of what they were supposed to learn, they actually learned. Those who supported the program, politically or monetarily, will have the opportunity to review evaluation results to decide whether to support the program again. Hill (2007) emphasizes the importance of assessing learning outcomes by polling students, faculty, and graduates to achieve depth and breadth in the reflection on program quality. Assessments may be qualitative, such as surveys or evaluation forms, or quantitative testing, which may pick up deficiencies.

A SWOT (strengths, weaknesses, opportunities, threats) analysis is a method of strategic planning that can be used both to generate ideas for a new curriculum and to evaluate curriculum reforms or to generate a list of curricular items for change (Henzi et al. 2007). The analysis permits choosing the most feasible items, given the resources available. A SWOT analysis can be used in any decision-making situation when a desired end-state (objective) has been defined. The aim of a SWOT analysis is to identify the key internal and external factors that are important to achieving the objective. In the case of curricula, the internal factors are the strengths and weaknesses internal to the curriculum, while the external factors are the opportunities and threats presented by the external environment to the curriculum.

TAKE-HOME POINTS

- **You need to explain up front why adults are learning something.**
- **Provide task-oriented instruction; adults learn through doing.**
- **Take into account a wide range of backgrounds; revel in having expertise.**
- **Adults are problem-solvers; use these skills.**
- **Adults learn best when the subject is of immediate use.**
- **Learning occurs at different cognitive levels.**
- **Objectives drive learning.**
- **Objectives may focus on several cognitive levels in a single exercise.**
- **Curricula are designed to achieve objectives.**
- **Assessment tests the learning of objectives.**
- **To be successful, doctors need to think analytically.**
- **Critical thinking is a learned skill fostered in medical school and on the wards.**
- **As a teacher, you will be expected to help others to think critically by encouraging questions, problem solving, gathering of accurate data, and assessment and evaluation of the evidence.**
- **Create interactive exercises that encourage critical thinking.**
- **Kern et al.'s six-step approach to curriculum development is logical, practical, and easy to follow.**
- **Carefully define the problem you want to solve.**
- **Objectives should be foolproof in their clarity.**
- **Different types of objective require different types of teaching exercise to achieve them.**
- **Evaluation must be built into the initial plans.**
- **A SWOT analysis may help you determine what curriculum change is most likely to succeed and is a good way to evaluate what you need to do to improve its chances of success.**

CHAPTER SIX

Assessing the Learner, Providing Feedback, Writing Evaluations and Recommendations

- *What type of question should I put on examinations? Is one type more valid than another?*
- *How do I make up good multiple-choice questions?*
- *When does an audience-response system improve an educational exercise?*
- *How should I prepare, if at all, for being an examiner in an objective structured clinical exam?*
- *How do I provide feedback to the student, resident, or fellow who is not performing well?*
- *How can I more quickly and efficiently write evaluations and recommendations?*

Preparing Your Learners for Assessment

Pangaro and McGahie (2005) note that assessment or evaluation should be fun, interesting, and challenging. Instead, assessment is viewed with fear, suspicion, and dread. Assessment is a big stick ready to strike down the poorly prepared. Exam hurdles are present at every step of medical education, and it is important to understand the principles of assessment (Friedman 2005). Shumway and Harden (2003) emphasize that assessment should be valid, reliable, practical, and have the desired impact on learning. Successful teachers make learners feel that they are expertly prepared for assessments and examinations.

Your job as a successful teacher is to prepare your students, residents, fellows, and colleagues for their exams. How do you do this? First, you need to know what the exams ask or test. Second, you need to include in your teaching plans the major concepts, facts, physical examination findings, and differential diagnosis findings your learners are expected to know. Spend money in your local university or medical school bookstore or order on-line exam books. Buy the same books that the examinees are studying and gear your course, curriculum, and postgraduate presentation to covering much of what you see is expected of them. Include whatever else you wish as content, but do cover what they are expected to know. This is not teaching to the test; this is teaching what the student is expected to know on a national basis. Third, recognize that students view these national tests as important hurdles they need to overcome for a medical degree and a specialty certification. Prepare your students well and you will have their undying gratitude. Fourth, understand that learners praise and respect teachers who help them prepare, but disrespect teachers who leave them unprepared. Fifth, as a top teacher, align your teaching objectives with national and local test expectations. Don't be a maverick. Emphasize that what you see is required knowledge in current tests and textbooks. You may not agree with all the content that is on the test, but it is foolhardy to disparage USMLE or internal medicine, surgery, and subspecialty board expectations to your learners.

Before testing any student, resident, or faculty member on your course objectives, make sure that your instructional objectives were clearly taught, reiterated, and reviewed. Do not test learners on something you mention only once during a course. Rather, focus on the many concepts, facts, pathology specimens, and x-ray findings that you did teach in more than one setting, such as in a tutorial and a small-group discussion or in a pathology laboratory and a lecture. Objectives for the course, small groups, tutorials, and pathology laboratories must be clear, up front, and emphasized. This is what you will test your learners on. You will feel no guilt when a student does poorly because you know that he or she did not follow directions or read the assignments as outlined. You know that the problem lies in the student's study habits or is associated with personal or health reasons. Following the above rule makes grading, potentially failing, or remediating students much more straightforward. Give a fair test based on objectives, and you can rest easy with what occurs during and after the exam. Give an exam that is not based on what you emphasized and reviewed, that focuses on new material or material not emphasized in class or in required readings, and you will find yourself wasting countless hours to remedy the aftermath and to explain to disgruntled students why you gave the test you did.

Remember that examinations are not traps for students or showcases for your brilliance, but a chance for you to prove that what you taught was learned and can be tested for factual knowledge, comprehension, application, analysis, synthesis, and integration. Too often, exam makers believe it is important to make the exam hard or complex enough to distinguish the best students or learners from the rest. I disagree. The purpose of an exam is to see whether important concepts, which were your key objectives, were understood and assimilated by the majority of students rather than the minority of students. You, as the course director, are not on display for how smart you are. You are on display as a maker of fair and clear tests that follow your teaching plan simply.

Exam strategies that I find hard to fathom are (1) using the test to distinguish which learner is able to go to new heights of problem solving in areas that were not discussed during your class, small session, or syllabus (this type of question could be used for extra credit), and (2) making the test so difficult, tricky, or complicated that learners who studied are uncertain whether they got the answers to the questions right or wrong. Examinations should be reinforcing, straightforward, not devious or obtuse; they should leave the learners who studied with a satisfying feeling that they could readily and confidently answer questions about the material. I have seen an otherwise good course and good course director get poor ratings after a "tricky" test. Students rebel against a course director who designs an exam to show how bright he or she is as an exam maker rather than designing a realistic instrument of what the course taught and emphasized. Put time into teaching your material well and let the exam flow from what you have emphasized and taught.

Traditional Types of Examination Questions

Paper-and-pencil tests are traditionally divided into two groups: objective response and constructed response. In the objective response, a student or learner chooses an answer from several alternatives. Little or no writing is needed. The three major types of objective test are multiple choice, true/false, and matching. Constructed-response questions require a written response and may be one-word answers (short-answer questions) or several pages of a handwritten essay.

Testing of skills and behaviors may be done in a simulation laboratory, an objective structured clinical examination (OSCE), a witnessed physical exam, or a clinical encounter. These tests of skills will be discussed later in this chapter.

Multiple-Choice Questions

Multiple-choice questions are the most commonly used type of test item that medical students, residents, fellows, and postgraduates will be asked to complete during their careers. Students are usually able to complete multiple-choice questions at a rate of one to two per minute. The USMLE, Step 1 and Step 2, Clinical Knowledge examination (CK), currently use multiple-choice tests exclusively, focusing on the one-best-answer items. The MDME has a Web site to explain constructing test questions for the basic and clinical sciences (www.nbme.org/about/itemwriting.asp). There are two types of multiple-choice question: type A has four to five response options for a single question item, while type R has two to ten items with five to twenty-six matching option responses (Gronlund 2006a; Fincher 2005). The important point for the medical teacher who is constructing this type of test item is the need to correlate tightly the objectives of the course being taught and the questions being asked. I am consistently amazed at teachers who ask multiple-choice questions about material that they never taught but somehow feel the students should know. Testing trivial facts is also a foolish idea. Angry and frustrated students will complain and mark you and your course down. If you did not teach or emphasize a concept or fact during your lecture, tutorial, or small-group session, do not put it on the midterm or final exam. If, on the other hand, you ask multiple-choice questions that cover content areas that you have singled out as important, relevant, and key to the field, then there is good validity to the multiple-choice question type of test. You will also have students praising you as a giver of fair tests.

Determine test questions by reviewing the major topics and subtopics. Identify the key points you have made. Construct your exam questions from declarative sentences containing the top principles or concepts you want students to remember. Well-written objectives are crucial to designing appropriate exam questions and to ensuring learner competence in the intended fields. Bloom et al. (1956) described six levels of increasingly complex learning: (1) knowledge or recall, (2) comprehension, (3) application, (4) analysis, (5) synthesis, and (6) evaluation. Collins (2006) notes that educators have simplified the levels to three broad categories, namely, (1) knowledge and recall, (2) comprehension and application, which means understanding and explaining in your own words both new and old knowledge, and (3) problem solving, which is defined as transferring existing knowledge to new situations.

Multiple-choice questions consist of a *stem,* which is the question, or an incomplete statement, and the *answers,* or alternatives to choose from. The stem is written first, as a complete sentence or question. The stem is frequently a clinical vignette. It should contain the following information:

- Patient's age and sex
- Presenting symptoms
- Pertinent history
- Pertinent physical exam
- Pertinent laboratory findings

A stem can incorporate diagrams, graphs, x-rays, and/or pathology slides. A stem should have all the relevant information but be kept as short as possible. The stem should not be used as a teaching opportunity, nor should it have extraneous information. Stems should not be "tricky" or difficult to read, because reading ability is not what is being tested. When application of knowledge is tested, then using stems containing vignettes of patient cases is helpful. The question or lead-in statement could be one of the following:

- Which of the following is the most likely diagnosis?
- Which is the most appropriate next step in treatment?
- Which is the most likely explanation of the patient's findings?

Avoid questions that have a lead-in such as:

Each of the following statements about _____ is correct except . . .
Which of the following statements about _____ is correct?

The test taker should be able to answer the question without having to look at the answer options.

The stem should be worded such that only one of the answers can be correct. Options for answers generally range from three to five alternatives. One answer is correct, and the rest are called distracters. It may be difficult to find more than four alternatives, or distracter answers, that appear plausible. Collins (2006) notes that the best distracters are (1) statements that are accurate but do not fully meet the requirements of the problem outlined, or (2) incorrect statements that seem right to the examinee. Each incorrect alternative should be plausible, but clearly incorrect. Distracters should be linked to one another and to the correct answer. For example, all the distracters could be diagnoses, tests, treatments, or prognoses. The distracters should be similar to the right answer in terms of grammar, length, and complexity. The examinee should not be able to figure out what the answer is by looking at the grammatical construction of the alternative answers. Thus, if the stem is plural or past tense, all the options should be plural or past tense.

Levels of Bloom's taxonomy of learning (knowledge, comprehension, application, analysis, and clinical reasoning or problem solving) can be checked with multiple-choice questions. The two highest levels of learning—synthesis and evaluation—are more easily tested by essay questions. In summary, the advantage of multiple-choice questions is that they are easy to grade and can check several levels of learning. The difficulty is that students can guess correctly at answers, the tests are hard to make up, and they primarily test recognition rather than recall.

In addition to linking the content of the questions to your educational objectives, Kemp, Morrison, and Ross (1994) recommend the following tips for making up multiple-choice questions: (1) decrease the length of the alternatives by moving as many words as possible to the stem, (2) design the stem so that it contains a complete thought and have the correct answer blend in with the distracters, giving all answers similar phrasing and length, (3) avoid the use of *always* and *never* as well as *all of the above* and *none of the above*, (4) phrase the question in a positive rather than a negative direction, (5) randomly select the position of the correct answer so that it is not always in the B or C position, (6) avoid, or at least define, abbreviations, acronyms, and eponyms, (7) place alternatives in a logical sequence, if possible, (8) do not have options in one item give away the correct answer to another question (this error in writing multiple-choice questions is called *cueing;* an option in one item provides a hint to the answer for another item), and (9) do not make one question "hinge" on another (students must know the answer to one question in order to answer another question).

Item discrimination is the percentage difference in correct responses between the top and bottom groups of students taking the test. An item with a discrimination of 60 percent or greater is considered a good item, while one with a discrimination of less than 19 percent is a low-discrimination item and should be revised.

Multiple-choice questions are evaluated for their reliability, validity, and resource intensiveness. *Reliability* refers to whether the item can be generalized; this means that the test score should be indicative of the score that the same student would receive on any other set of relevant items. *Validity* refers to whether a test measures what it says it is measuring. *Resource intensiveness* is the cost of constructing the multiple-choice exams. While multiple-choice questions are easy, objective, and reliable to grade, they are difficult to write. Faculty may benefit from a one-hour workshop on writing multiple-choice questions. It may be useful to have a meeting to make up the test. Each test writer is asked to send in sample questions ahead of time, and all questions are then read aloud or shown on a screen or blackboard to determine which are the best. Let someone who did not write any of the exam questions read them. Ask that person to put him- or herself in the student's position. Questions should get at problem-solving skills, not just factual knowledge.

True/False Questions

If you wish to use true/false test questions, the content of your educational exercises must be in a form that permits you to ask this type of question (generally factual) (Gronlund, 2006b). The advantages are that true/false questions are relatively easy to write and easy to grade. However, they test recognition of facts, permit guessing, and focus on testing the two lowest levels of learning in Bloom's taxonomy: knowledge and comprehension. Tips from Kemp, Morrison, and Ross (1994) for creating this type of question are: (1) be sure that the statement is totally true or totally false, (2) communicate only one thought or idea in a true/false statement, and (3) use this type of question infrequently, given the high percentage of guessing.

Matching Columns

Matching columns ask the learner to identify relationships between a list of items in one column and answers in another column, preferably all on the same page, to minimize turning pages back and forth (Gronlund, 2006b). Uses of the matching columns include testing for definitions and terms, dates and events, functions and parts, and achievements and people. The big advantage of this type of testing is the large amount of material that can be evaluated in a relatively small space and the opportunity to ask questions that cross disciplines (Fincher 2005). Tips for creating matching columns by Kemp, Morrison, and Ross (1994) are: (1) limit the number of items to six or seven, (2) limit the length of the question to a word, phrase, or brief sentence, and (3) give one or two additional distracters to decrease the probability of guessing.

Short-Answer and Essay Questions

The main advantage of the constructed-response question (short-answer or essay) is that learners can express their knowledge and problem-solving ability in their own words. The major problem is the inability to obtain reliable grading for these types of question.

Short-answer questions are also known as "fill in the blanks." The answer can be a word, phrase, symbol, number, or complete sentence. Bloom's taxonomy levels of knowledge or recall, comprehension or application, can be graded. The questions must be unambiguous to minimize subjective scoring (Schuwirth and van der Vleuten 2005). Two problems are associated with this type of question: (1) it is difficult to phrase the question so that only one response is right, and (2) learners may have spelling difficulties, so it is not always clear to the grader whether an answer is correct or not. The short answer is less subject to guessing and can test a broad range of knowledge. Gronlund's (2006b) rules for writing short-answer questions include: (1) stating the item so that only a single brief answer is possible, (2) using a direct question if possible, (3) having only one blank (this is best), and (4) putting the blank at the end of the statement.

Essay questions give the student a large degree of freedom. Gronlund (2006b, 115) notes that, in the essay question, students are "free to decide how to approach the problem, what factual information to use, how to organize the answer, and what degree of emphasis to give each aspect of the response. Thus, the essay question is especially useful for measuring the ability to organize, integrate, and express ideas." This utility distinguishes the essay from the selection-type test or short-answer test. Essays are not particularly useful, on the other hand, for sampling content; scoring is subjective, difficult, and unreliable; good writing ability and bluffing may mask weak answers.

Essays can be restricted or unrestricted. The restricted-response essay question places limits on the quantity written by indicating that the answer should *list, name,* or *define.* Other limits may be given, such as the number of pages or words. This type of essay can be constructed and scored more readily than the unrestricted essay, but it does not permit the teacher to assess the ability to organize, integrate, and create new connections with the material to the extent that the unrestricted essay does. The extended-response unrestricted essay gives more freedom to create, integrate, and evaluate ideas. The major problem in the unrestricted essay is evaluating the answers with reliability.

Students who write well or can bluff may do better than they should, while students who are poor spellers or write illegibly or make grammatical errors are unlikely to receive as much credit as those who are good writers and spellers and who write legibly.

Essay questions should be designed to measure a well-defined outcome. You may wish to indicate to the learners the criteria on which you will judge the essay (e.g., strength of differential diagnosis, relevant background material, logical analysis of the problem, management of the problem, and recommendations for therapeutic interventions). In your essay question, use words such as *compare, contrast, describe,* and *explain* to encourage students to demonstrate the complex connections and interconnections they have made. It is preferable, according to Gronlund (2006b), to give no choice in answering the essay questions, but rather to give all students the same questions to answer. This gives you as a teacher a better opportunity to compare students. Give students enough time to answer questions; the test is not a test of speedwriting.

Grading essays is plagued by subjectivity. Gronlund (2006b) makes several excellent suggestions regarding the grading of essays: (1) evaluate the answers for the specific outcome you have set up (ignore the writing and spelling), (2) use model answers as a guide to scoring points on restricted-response questions, (3) for extended-response questions make up criteria for quality and judge each essay on these criteria (divide the students' exams into separate piles: excellent, good, fair, and poor responses), (4) consider grading all students' exams for one essay question before going on to the next question, (5) make your evaluations less subjective by masking the students' names, (6) have two, or more than two, graders be responsible for grading each answer in order to check the independence and reliability of the grading system.

Preclinical Testing, Quizzes, and Final Examinations

Creating exam questions is hard work. Because of this, be sure to save all exam questions for make-up tests and subsequent quizzes and final exams. Once several years have passed, these old exams are excellent sources of questions.

Quizzes during a preclinical course are useful barometers of student learning. The quizzes, which let you know if your students understand and remember, generally comprise ten multiple-choice questions, each with four or five possible answers and one best answer. I give one or two quizzes during a two-and-a-half-week course. I choose facts and concepts that I have emphasized more than once. If a pancreatic pseudocyst is mentioned in lecture and a mini-case session as well as in the weekly review session, I feel good about asking students to define or identify a pancreatic pseudocyst. On the other hand, if I have mentioned pseudocyst only in small-group session and not in my review session or in a lecture or a tutorial, I would not use it as an exam item. I know that during their surgery rotation, gastroenterology elective, medicine clerkship, and radiology elective clerkship, students will be asked about pancreatic pseudocysts, so I emphasize their origin and appearance during the course.

Final examinations summarize what the student is taking away from your course. The final examination I create may be a composite of multiple-choice questions, short-answer questions, and short essays or solely multiple-choice questions. Essay grading is easy when the student is right on the mark. However, it is hard when the student has some correct and some incorrect statements. Then intergrader variability may occur and the grading is less reliable. Make up the answer key before the exam day because your exam graders need it to begin their work. I ask the medical school to provide a classroom, sandwiches, cookies, and soft drinks for several graders on the day of the exam. Because the multiple-choice questions are graded by a machine or by administrators, I have only one grading session for faculty who wish to see how the short-answer and short-essay grading is done and want to grade several exams. After this grading session, I grade all the remaining exams for consistency and double check all the exams graded by others for consistency before I hand them in.

Within two weeks, all medical school and dental school student exams have been graded and passed back to students with the detailed, annotated answer key, if essays are involved, or the correct-answer key, if solely multiple-choice questions were used.

Exam Failures, Proctoring, and Accommodation of Disability

After grading all the exams, I pull out the lowest-scoring exams and reread them to see if I made an error. If I correct any errors in grading, I then reread the potentially failing exams carefully for content and understanding. Does this student know enough to pass the exam even though the exam score is low? If multiple answers are well below the minimum standard for comprehension and factual knowledge, I will fail this student; he or she will be given back the exam and the answer key. A make-up exam with new questions will be scheduled for several weeks later. A significant problem is the student who fails the exam and wishes to take the make-up exam within one to two weeks, but then fails it again. To avoid this potential major problem, I personally meet with each failing student to find out why he or she did not study or was distracted. The reasons are usually a personal or social problem (such as a family or personal illness) or excessive involvement with extracurricular activities, research, summer job, or grant activities. I have given a short review course for one student who failed the course final exam and make-up exam due to excessive extracurricular activities. After the private review course, the student did well. I put in a lot of effort to help this student but was pleased when he finally learned the material.

Several years ago, during parents' weekend at my son's college, I sat in on an evolutionary biology course. An exam was given during the latter part of the class. I was surprised to see the instructor walk out of the class after handing out the exam. Because no formal honor code exists in my medical school, as it does at my son's college, I proctor the quizzes and final exam with my teaching fellow. We sit at a table in the front of the room and answer questions from students. When enough students ask the same question, I will call out to the class a clarification of the confusing question. This clarification is frequently helpful to the entire class. If students are retaking the final exam due to illness or a failure, I sit in the small room with them to answer any questions that may come up.

Be alert to the students in the class who have a disability. Accommodation will be arranged for them through the disabilities office at the medical school. Over the years, I have had students with physical disabilities and learning disabilities. Students have taken the test on a computer in a private room and others have taken extra time with a paper test. Depending on the disability, students may ask to take an oral exam rather than a written exam. I have given an oral exam to a student with severe dyslexia. The student knew the material and passed the test easily. Oral exams, in general, are not very reliable, due to the biases of the examiner.

Outcome-based Education

As I listened to Dr. Robert Alpern and Dr. Sharon Long describe their new report for the AAMC and Howard Hughes Medical Institute (HHMI), entitled "Scientific Foundations for Future Physicians," at the 2009 Annual AAMC Meeting's Council of Academic Societies Annual Meeting Program, I was reminded of outcome-based education in medicine, which focuses on what competencies physicians should possess at the end of medical school (Harden 2002; Harden, Crosby, and Davis 1999). The AAMC/HHMI report recommends that premedical education, instead of being a list of static required courses, be a series of innovative and interdisciplinary science curricula leading to a dynamic set of measurable competencies.

Outcome-based education has been embraced by schools in Australia, South Africa, Malaysia, Chile, the United Kingdom, and the United States (Davis and Harden 2003). W. G. Spady (1994, 12) defined outcome-based education as "clearly focusing and organizing everything in an educational system around what is essential for all students to be able to do successfully at the end of their experiences." In 1996, Brown University Medical School began to use a competency-based curriculum with a defined set of competency requirements, which all medical students who expect to graduate must show they have achieved (Smith and Dollase 1999). A faculty member determines if an individual student has reached competence by using a performance-based method of assessment. Dannefer and Henson (2007) published the Cleveland Clinic Lerner College of Medicine's Portfolio approach to competency-based assessment, with an online Portfolio for each student, which provides a method for collecting and managing the various types of assessment results from multiple different parts of the curriculum. The AAMC has assisted efforts for outcome-based education with the publication of a monograph (www.hhmi.org/grants/sffp.html) that defines the qualities, skills, and knowledge that medical students should have at graduation and lists learning objectives to achieve these competency-based goals.

Audience-Response Systems

Audience-response systems permit students to respond and interact with the teacher via hand-held remote keypads that note the respondents' answers and transmit them to a central computer in the room (Caldwell 2007; Wood 2004). The answers can be immediately tabulated and shown on a projection screen to the entire class for discussion.

Why use this technology? The audience-response system permits you to poll your students to see if they have understood concepts, to obtain student opinions on a differential diagnosis and the correct pharmacological intervention, and to increase interactions among a lecture hall full of students. The technology involves *keypads* or *clickers,* which are small transmitters that generally have a ten-digit numerical keypad with a power switch, a send button, and function keys that allow text entry (Caldwell 2007; Wood 2004). Current systems are bidirectional, with the clicker sending a signal and indicating whether it has been received. They are wireless and use radiofrequency signals. One of the standard principles is that each clicker has a unique signal, so the answer from each student can be identified and recorded. When the entire class has completed its answers, the results are displayed, often in the form of a histogram. The audience-response system couples a receiver unit with an ordinary classroom computer and projection system. The software used to create and administer the questions is not more complex than that for displaying slides. The teacher has grading tools in the software, which permit different points to be allotted to correct versus incorrect answers. Clickers or keypads can be used in large and small classes and in group settings.

The questions are usually written before class as part of the class plan. Generally, two to five questions are asked during a fifty-minute time slot. Types of question include collecting votes after a debate; assessing student preparation and students' understanding of the lecture material, quizzes, and tests; practice problems, for review at the end of lecture; and for conducting experiments. We have used audience response successfully in a preclinical setting to prepare students for the boards. Multiple-choice questions using a typical national board format are put up on a screen or handed out as exam questions. Students love the anonymity of the response and the quick feedback, focused on understanding the material. Cain (2008) reported that pharmacy students found that strategically placed questions in physiological chemistry/molecular biology course lectures helped keep their attention, while the teachers were able to adapt their lectures to stress areas that were identified through the audience-response system as being deficient.

Most review articles show that the clickers increase student participation in class and increase attendance, when clicker scores account for part of the student's grade. Audience-response systems decrease the time for content coverage in lecture, but the decreased coverage appears to be offset by improved student comprehension, the instructor's ability to assess in real time whether the pacing of the course is on the mark, and improved instructor awareness of student difficulties. Students generally enjoy clickers and feel that teachers who use them are more caring and knowledgeable about the students' needs. Students enjoy the anonymity in answering questions, the reinforcement of learning, and the ability to compare their standing in the answers with that of the rest of the class. Negative student comments focus on the cost of the clickers, the possibility of losing the clicker and having to pay for it, and anxiety as to whether a score, if it will be part of the grade, was properly counted. Instructors like the clickers because they increase class discussions, but they dislike the cost, any glitches that occur technically, and the time necessary to address questions concerning alternative answers. In addition, it takes time and practice to develop questions, but the questions can often be reused. The only rule for making up questions is that each question address a learning goal.

Clickers are powerful and flexible tools for teaching a variety of subjects at every level. They appear to increase attendance and can promote student accountability. Large classes benefit from the stimulation and motivation. However, the jury is still out as to whether they improve retention of the material.

Objective Structured Clinical Examination

Harden and Gleeson (1979) introduced the term *objective structured clinical examination* (OSCE) to refer to five- to thirty-minute examination stations at which students must demonstrate specific clinical skills. Key features include all students being examined on the same tasks and graded with a standardized scoring sheet. OSCE is the main performance-based skills exam that medical students will be repeatedly exposed to during the course of their four years. The format is flexible and can be adapted to meet diverse groups' needs. The big issue in this type of exam is reliability (Marks and Humphrey-Murto 2005). Turner and Dankoski (2008) review the positives and negatives of the OSCE and focus on the issues that need to be addressed when designing and planning an OSCE.

Studies have shown that, with training, the standardized patients, interrater agreement, exam reliability, and standardization across multiple testing sites can be brought into a reasonable range. Medical school OSCE exams may range from ten to twelve stations to twenty-five to thirty stations, depending on resources and personnel. The length of the stations is frequently from five to eight minutes, with two minutes for feedback and one minute to move to the next station. Checklists used vary from those that note whether an exam has been performed to those that measure communication skills. The checklist for the former may be simple, with a check indicating the correct performance of the exam and the absence of a check indicating that this did not occur, for whatever reason. The communication-skill list may take the form of a Likert scale from 1 to 5, where a range of ability can be expressed for the different categories.

OSCE uses standardized patients, as does the USMLE, Step 2, Clinical Skills examination (CS). Standardized patients (paid actors) are helpful to give students the patient's point of view. However, a systematic review of the ways in which standardized patients are trained to give feedback to students revealed that there are no clear standards or methods. Rather, the feedback is "heterogeneous" and seems to "lack a solid scientific basis" (Bokken et al. 2009, 207).

Videotaped sessions of students interacting with standardized patients can be reviewed with the student to obtain a full 360-degree evaluation, with several different perspectives. This type of evaluation is time-consuming, but receiving this information about his or her performance may be rewarding for the student.

Students rotate from station to station, asking history questions and performing physical examinations on standardized patients. As a faculty member, you will be assigned to a station. Your recruitment probably occurred months earlier, and you may have forgotten your assignment. Often you will be acquainted with the station shortly before your role is to begin on the day of the exam. The acquaintance session is one to which all examiners that morning or afternoon are invited. Generally, food is available, but I try to eat beforehand so that I can focus on my duties as examiner immediately. It is good to have a cup of coffee or tea to bring into the station if it is a long afternoon session, so you don't flag in your enthusiasm and energy. If the station objectives, scenario, and notes are not sent to you ahead of time, ask for them. I do not like teaching surprises and like to prepare ahead of time. I bring along visual aids in the form of library atlases or diagrams to help the students understand what they might have missed and how they could have approached or diagnosed the problem. I also have a physical diagnosis text with bookmarks indicating useful diagrams and patient pictures with the organ of interest highlighted (LeBlond, DeGowin, and Brown 2004).

Arrive at the OSCE early enough to visit the station before you host it. Familiarize yourself with the buzzer or bell that will indicate the need for the students to stop, to move, and to start a new station. Learn how to use the stopwatch, if it is available, as an additional safeguard to help you stay on time. It is preferable to see your actual station so that you know where to stand or sit to be most effective and not in the way; you need an accurate view of what is taking place to be an impartial judge. At the station, begin to visualize yourself examining students. Introduce yourself to the standardized patient and get to know his or her style. This standardized patient will be evaluating the student. Understanding his or her perspective may help you to anticipate how he or she will grade the student. Familiarize yourself with the checklist sheet you will be filling out. Complete all the paperwork you can before you begin (name, phone number, e-mail address, etc.) because, at the end, monitors will be requesting the finalized paperwork almost immediately. Whatever happens, complete the checklist evaluations as you see each student. Do not leave anything undone until the end. Too many students pass through your station to believe that you will remember to write a note or change a grade after the student has left and another has started into your station. At the breaks, be sure to finalize any opinion surveys and fill in any last-minute items on the required forms. Your paperwork will be due immediately after your time slot is over. Do not be tardy, or you risk your students' evaluations being lost in the monitors' rush for the door. Monitors, who have been at their stations all day, try to finish promptly and leave their grueling tasks. Your evaluations cannot be redone, if they are mislaid, because they are long, detailed checklists.

As noted above, I prepare ahead each time I am an OSCE preceptor. First, I read and reread the scenario and the objectives. Then I decide on what may be important points to emphasize. For instance, I generally proctor the abdominal exam station, where each student has both a history to take and a physical exam of the abdomen to perform. The whole station takes about fifteen minutes, including feedback from both the standardized patient and me, the attending preceptor. Before the OSCE, I study the classic history questions to ask the patient presenting with an acute abdomen, and I focus on a few that are frequently forgotten or not well understood. I study the abdominal exam, visualizing the steps (such as percussion and palpation of the liver and spleen) that often give students trouble. I also review the maneuvers to elicit the presence of ascites.

I find books in the medical library or in my own teaching collection that have diagrams to help students visualize the proper placement of hands for the various abdominal exam maneuvers. I bring these books into the station in my wheeling suitcase to show during the five-minute feedback session if a student has had trouble with the exam portion of the station. Once prepared with teaching points and visuals, I know that I will give practical and useful feedback to each student concerning the history and/or physical exam. Illustrating specific points of the underlying anatomy with an anatomical atlas or of the physical exam with excellent diagrams has worked well to help students gain or solidify knowledge about the abdominal exam. I find that students appreciate learning the abdominal exam through illustrations showing how to place their hands, position their body, or correctly drape the patient at the abdominal exam station.

What do you do when the student starts off completely wrong, such as approaching the bed or stretcher for the abdominal examination from the wrong (left) side of the body? When I first began as an OSCE examiner, I wanted to tell the student immediately that he or she was on the wrong side of the bed and should start over. I saw the problem as awful and obvious. However, I did not do that because I realized that this is the student's chance to make this type of basic mistake and be corrected for it without major consequences. Perhaps the correction will fix the right way of examining the abdomen in the student's mind forever. As the years have gone on, I have become more and more aware that the OSCE is an opportunity for each student to learn and improve on the spot. Few students fail, and those who do receive much-appreciated remediation. I am calmer about the mistakes I see. The OSCE will let both student and teacher know that there are rough edges to be rounded off after the exam by practice. I no longer agonize over having few items checked on a twenty-five-item score sheet. The student will get help and improve. It is not a do-or-die situation. Rather, the OSCE is an opportunity to dispassionately see what a wide range of budding clinical skills are present in each student class. Some students are so proficient that they should be the examiners; others are so deficient that you wonder where they have been during the sessions that gave practice on detailed history taking and physical exams. I have taken the poor students' performance as a signal to give more opportunities for practice after our introduction to the abdominal exam session. Each student is given the opportunity to do the exam twice on two different people (one a fellow student and one a mystery patient) during the introductory teaching session. Each student is offered longitudinal follow-up in a doctor's office to perform abdominal exams on outpatients to practice the skills he or she has learned.

Occasionally, I have found a standardized patient whom I felt was unfair in his or her summary comments to a student about the interaction between the two of them that I had observed. This has occurred particularly with overconfident students or quiet, unassertive students. In these cases, after the standardized patient has finished his or her comments, I will gently modify, or shift the emphasis of, the standardized patient's comments before I give my own feedback on the specifics of history and the physical exam. I prefer to alter the tone of the interaction evaluation immediately to soften the blow of a harsh judgment I feel is unwarranted. On rare occasions, I have seen an arrogant and defensive student in an OSCE station approach the patient in a patronizing manner or argue about the evaluations being given by the standardized patient or the preceptor. This student does need to hear loudly, clearly, and immediately that his or her approach is unacceptable to both patient and examiners.

Feedback

Principles of Effective Feedback

Ende (1983) noted that feedback sets the stage for improvement. When feedback fails, it is often because of the recipient's anger, defensiveness, or failure to see the utility of the observations and suggestions offered. Teachers need to work with the learners as allies. Bing-You and Trowbridge (2009) noted that feedback may fail if the learner's capacity for self-reflection (metacognition) about his or her thoughts and feelings is limited. Adequate metacognitive ability is necessary for the feedback to be interpreted appropriately by the learner. Otherwise learners may deny or discount negative feedback.

Feedback should deal with specific details of diagnosis and management. Personality traits that cannot be changed should not be included. The focus should be on the decisions made and the thinking behind them. Don't fail to point out correctable mistakes. Use language that is precise, objective, and encourages change. Feedback on strengths and weaknesses given on a regular basis to trainees or students is called *formative assessment,* as opposed to *summative assessment,* which determines who passes and who fails. The summative assessment also indicates whether a certain standard for learning has been reached (McAleer and Hesketh 2003).

Preclinical Feedback

Preclinical feedback sessions during a course lasting several weeks are usually scheduled for ten-minute intervals. Design a feedback grid with times, dates, and cell phone numbers for a midcourse feedback session (fig. 6.1). The cell phone numbers are helpful if you need to contact students who fail to show up for a feedback session or if you recognize that you will be unavoidably late and will need to reschedule the session.

	7:00 a.m.	7:10 a.m.	7:20 a.m.	7:30 a.m.	7:40 a.m.	7:50 a.m.
Tuesday, March 17						
Friday, March 20						
Tuesday, March 24						

Figure 6.1. **Student Feedback Schedule for Faculty Members**
Fill in this grid with each student's name and phone number on the first day of
the course, tutorial, small-group meeting, or seminar. Remind a student of an
appointment the day before with a phone call and voice mail message to the cell
phone number to minimize tardiness or a student's forgetting the appointment.

Feedback sessions run smoothly if you, in fact, have done your homework
and collected the appropriate concrete material. How do you collect this material? After each tutorial or small-group session, write out comments about
each student and your impressions of each student's contribution to the group
process and knowledge on a log or paper designated for feedback (see fig. 6.2).
Focus on the student's preparation, participation, quality of the information
and clarity of thinking, types of question asked, ability to teach others in the
group, and personal interactions with group members. Refresh your memory
with your recorded notes before you begin each student's session. Do not show
your collected note sheet, if possible, to the student. However, do cite from
memory "chapter and verse" of the student's contributions to the tutorial or
seminar. Specific dates and connections are both useful and believable.

Have a plan for your part of the interaction, but be willing to scrap the
plan if the learner wants to tell you something about the situation or his or
her own perspective to help you understand his or her side of the story. I viv-
idly remember the student who came for tutorial feedback many years ago.
She had missed several sessions, owing, I thought, to illness, and she seemed
down and disinterested. When we met, I opened the conversation and asked
how she felt she had done, knowing full well that she had been disengaged
and had not done very well in tutorial. I was horrified to hear her calmly say
that her father had been murdered; that is why she had been away. Her dis-

Student	Tues., March 24	Thurs., March 26	Fri., March 27

Figure 6.2. **Faculty Comments on Student Participation**
Note, on a daily basis, what each student did or said to move the tutorial to a better understanding of the science, physiology, pathophysiology, and cultural, racial, ethnic, and socioeconomic aspects of the case. Did the student ask a question, diagram a mechanism on the blackboard, bring in a reference, lead the group in a different direction with new knowledge, or encourage another student's entering into the discussion? Having these notes will make the individual feedback session and the final evaluation easier.

engagement was a result of this terrible tragedy, which she had kept hidden from her classmates and me until I asked her something about her perspective. After this episode, I changed my attitude toward feedback. Feedback is a great way to get to know the person you may be negatively or positively evaluating. What he or she says during this short focused time may change dramatically how you judge him or her in the future. It is important to keep an open mind as you go into a feedback session, especially one in which you expect to give a negative evaluation.

Tutorial Evaluation

Tutorial evaluations, while qualitative, are the single best measure of a preclinical student's preparation and participation in medical schools where the first two years record pass/fail grades. Issues of professionalism, personal style of learning, leadership qualities, creativity and clarity of thought, ability to draw concepts, ability to be a team player—all will show up in the tutorial. How do you remember each student and what he or she did? How do you write an individual personalized assessment? A foolproof way is to make a grid with each day of the tutorial on it and enough spaces for tutees' names (fig. 6.2). Before you start teaching, put each student's name into the comment grid and begin religiously noting the accomplishments and the role in the tutorial for each tutee, using one to three phrases or sentences for each tutorial contact. The grid allows for a telegraphic style to record each student's contribution.

Be cautious about putting negative comments in a final preclinical evaluation unless you have given specific, clear feedback about a negative behavior (such as coming in late repeatedly or being consistently unprepared) and the behavior has not changed as a result of your feedback. Your negative feedback to a student should be documented in your records after your oral feedback session with this student, along with the student's comments, reply, or rebuttal. Because tutorial evaluations are frequently used verbatim for dean's letters, carefully construct your comments and read them over out loud before you send them to the course director. In the tutorial evaluation paragraph, I comment on the level of preparation and participation of each student, with specific instances of things the student did to ensure the tutorial's success as a learning exercise by bringing in information, drawing concepts, leading the discussion, or asking questions for clarification. In addition, I describe the student's ability to lead the group or to function as a good team player. I end by summarizing the student's overall performance in one sentence.

Clinical Feedback

Allow at least a fifteen-minute time interval for giving clinical feedback. Ende (1983) noted that feedback is information used to make adjustments in reaching a goal. Feedback is formative and free of judgment, while evaluations are summative because they are given at the end of a rotation, after any changes can be made. Feedback is frequently scarce, and that may be because it is difficult to obtain the firsthand observations on which to base feedback. Teachers also worry that negative feedback will damage the student-teacher or resident-teacher relationship and hurt the teacher's popularity. These fears may lead to talking around a problem or using unclear terminology about what is meant. The student may reinforce the teacher's avoidance because he or she is worried about a negative evaluation.

Feedback is important in clinical medicine to correct mistakes and change performance. Students may learn only after the clerkship is finished that their performance was considered sub par. Medical students' progress in the clinical arena should be evaluated frequently to be sure the students are performing at an appropriate level. It is preferable to evaluate at the bedside rather than in a conference room. Go to the bedside and observe the student taking a history or performing a physical exam. This will give you a much better idea of the clinical skills than just listening to the student present a case and introduce the patient to you on rounds. For residents, it is the same. The resident can improve with specific targeted feedback, based not on hearsay but on direct observations. However, few teaching attending physicians take the time to sit down with the resident to go over how he or she has performed, using specific instances of witnessed optimal behavior or suboptimal behavior to launch the discussion.

A key principle is for feedback to be based on what the student, resident, fellow, and teacher have previously agreed on as the goals for the educational sessions they will share. Perhaps the commonest mistake I make in this area occurs when I am a clinical attending. I frequently fail to distinctly articulate the goals that I expect the learners to attain. I do not make sure that the students, residents, and fellows agree with stated clear goals and expectations that I silently have for rounds, presentations, and follow-ups. Failing to articulate goals sets me up for a difficult time at the end of the rotation, when feedback must occur. How can I complain when the fellow never understood my expectations? Make feedback easier and less painful by having ground rules that you announce on the first day of your attending duties. Your evaluations will be based on your learners' adhering to or exceeding the guidelines for performance you have set forth in your introductory speech. Recognizing your own distaste for feedback is fine as long as it propels you to set up a structure that cannot fail you in this awkward but essential area.

From the first day, let each student, resident, or fellow know that he or she will have a mid-rotation and a final feedback session with you. These can be as short as five minutes or as long as an hour, if problems arise. Jot down a phrase, word, or grade each day in categories such as communication skills, preparation, participation, clinical bedside skills, physical exam skills, progress-note capabilities, accuracy and completeness of follow-up information. Keep this note card or grid in a prominent place for you to access on a daily basis or remind yourself at the end of the day to evaluate the student, resident, or fellow's performance before going to bed. Keeping notes makes all the difference between dreading the feedback session and welcoming it as an opportunity to show what data you have gathered and how it stacks up against your stated expectations.

How it comes together is another issue. How do you weigh various aspects of a physician-in-training's performance? How do you weigh great presentations and skilled clinical exam skills when the fellow, resident, or student has been missing in action and unavailable by page when he or she was needed to do a lumbar puncture? Was it a simple matter of a dead battery? Was it a miscommunication? Was it a sign that this talented student has a veneer of clinical interest but beneath the surface, desires to be free of the draining and time-consuming medical teamwork? Does this person's long-term plans make entrepreneurship rather than clinical medicine his or her preferred career? Is he or she working on deals or research projects to the detriment of clinical work? While it is essential to teach and model professional behavior in medical school, Papadakis et al. (2005) demonstrated that it is equally important to identify and give immediate feedback on unprofessional behavior so that interventions and remediation can be tried.

Because clinical evaluations are important as a means of changing behavior, skills, and attitudes, base what you say about a student or resident on concrete evidence. Having "chapter and verse" about the clinical skills you have witnessed is the easiest and best way to make feedback a useful time for you and the learner. Specifics of great clinical care or of shoddy care, which you believe you will remember, are frequently forgotten by the end of the rotation, when the evaluation is due. The evaluation form generally asks you to indicate the date of the feedback session. Make sure you record details of the feedback session, such as the date, time, length of session, and what was said, for future reference. The student, resident, or fellow may come to you for a recommendation or may question the grade he or she is given. You may be called in to discuss with the clerkship director or with the learner your evaluation and why you gave it. Save your specific comments regarding observations and interactions on paper or in an online folder that you designate as your feedback folder. This will avoid future problems if the learner disputes the evaluation.

In your feedback session, begin by asking how things are going. After the learner has finished discussing his or her feelings, indicate your comments about the clinical skills he or she has displayed. If the skills are superlative, then the rest of the time may be left for questions or for the student's asking you about career direction or other issues. If you wish the student to change or alter a behavior to reach a goal of improved performance, focus on one or two things that can be changed, such as poorly organized or overly long presentations, inadequate physical exams, missing laboratory and radiological data, or snap judgments made on inadequate data. Describe rather than judge what you have seen. Use specifics of date, time, and place to objectify your comments. If you have subjective comments to make about your or others' perceptions of the learner, make sure you label the feedback as subjective rather than objective. Focus on the learners' decisions and actions rather than on trying to interpret, assume, or guess why the learner has behaved in a certain way. Point the learner in the direction of a solution within his or her grasp for the problem you have identified.

Challenges to any feedback session are your own feelings about the learner, the feedback and the possibility for change, his or her defensiveness, inadequate time and observation to know for sure if this is his or her best performance. If there are cognitive concerns, then a referral to a specialist for testing may be in the learner's best interest. Always indicate that you are there to help solve the problem and will be an advocate.

Ende's (1983) guidelines for giving feedback are helpful. His key points are that it should:

1. be undertaken with the teacher and trainee working as allies, with common goals.
2. be well timed and expected.

3. be based on first-hand data.
4. be regulated in quantity and limited to behaviors that are remediable.
5. be phrased in descriptive, nonjudgmental language.
6. deal with specific performances, not generalizations.
7. offer subjective data, labeled as such.
8. deal with decisions and actions, rather than assumed intentions or interpretations.

Writing Evaluations and Recommendations

Writing evaluations is easy once you have two things: the data and the form. Start by obtaining a copy of the form that you will be expected to fill out for each student, resident, or fellow at the beginning of the rotation. Read it twice to make sure you know the criteria you will be expected to comment on. I dislike being asked to comment on a trait, characteristic, or skill that I have given no thought to during the rotation because I did not realize it was on the evaluation form. I feel as if I am guessing rather than being fair to the learner by having a thoughtful evaluation mentality. Be ready to offer a solution or detail the improvements made after initial negative feedback has been given. If major problems have arisen with professionalism, the form is not the place where the discussion should first appear. Rather, you should alert the chair or the head of the clerkship as soon as the problem surfaces. The form should indicate progress in areas that were identified as weak or needing remediation. If you feel that you had the student, resident, or fellow for too short an interval to evaluate performance, indicate this on the online or paper form and do not fill in the check boxes or complete the evaluation.

When I interviewed for the position of associate master of the Oliver Wendell Holmes Society, I was asked by Dr. Augustus White III, the master of the society, whether I enjoyed writing recommendation letters. I said I did, and this was true. It is fun to recommend people for positions, awards, and scholarships. I like helping those who have done well get benefit from letters I write on their behalf. In the associate master position, which is being an advisor to medical school students in their preclinical and clinical years, I write many recommendation letters. The solution to making it easy to write these letters is to have a template in your mind for the letter's organization. Then you fill in the blanks from the student's, resident's, fellow's, or faculty member's curriculum vitae (CV). The second way to make letter writing easy is to interview the person you are writing about to get your facts straight and to gain his or her perspective on what the major contributions have been. How does this person see his or her leadership potential? What activities indicate that he or she is a leader? Often the applicant has forgotten to list all accomplishments on the CV, but if questioned about leadership skills, volunteer activities, or even presentations and publications, will come up with things that are important nonetheless.

I dictate the majority of my letters into a Dictaphone. Be careful to keep checking that your words are registering. My assistant or I type shorter letters. I may dictate a short recommendation to my administrator if the letter must go off immediately. I tell each applicant at the end of the interview when he or she can expect that I will dictate the letter and approximately when my administrator will type the dictation. I encourage the applicant to work with my administrator to see the letter to completion. I have learned to set a time limit for the dictation of a recommendation letter (one hour maximum). The dictation time is separate from the initial interview time, which usually averages one hour. Occasionally an hour and a half may be needed, if the applicant has many honors, research or leadership accomplishments, or global health activities. I usually dictate letters at a specific time on a specific day of the week (Sunday evenings). This system works for me. I batch the recommendation letter writing so it all gets done in a prompt and relatively organized fashion.

I make copies for my administrator of all CV materials given to me; if I lose a copy, my administrator has the original or she has the e-mail with CV attachment that the student sent to me. I also send my administrator e-mail with all information about the deadline, Web site link for graduate schools of education, business, government, and public health. Some forms are presented as online links to complex forms for other degree programs, for which you may be asked to comment on such areas as skill in quantitative or mathematical techniques. If you are not sure, you may wish to ask the candidate if he or she took math or statistics in college and how he or she did in terms of grades. In addition, you may use the MCAT scores as helpful indicators of skills. At the end of the check boxes, give your overall impression in a few sentences. Be kind, gracious, but honest.

My administrators are kept aware of letters that need to be completed and the deadline by e-mail or voice mail. The administrators and I determine the urgency of the deadline and place each applicant in the queue of letters to be dictated, with the recommendation deadline as the first priority. I encourage the applicant to contact my administrator more than once, if necessary, to ensure that the recommendation letter will be completed on time. With this well-oiled system in place, my administrators and I can safely advertise to students, fellows, and faculty that we have never missed a deadline for a letter of recommendation. This puts the requestor's mind at ease, knowing that the letter of recommendation will go out on time even though he or she may have to do some prodding. Reminders from my administrator are important for getting letters finished when many other deadlines are competing for my attention. Recommendation letters can easily sink to the bottom of the work pile unless you have a strong organizational system for getting them done. Students, residents, fellows, and peers respect faculty who write great letters of recommendation and send them off on time.

Susan Whalley (2000, 5) notes in her book on writing recommendations that "writing a recommendation requires vitality, concentration and knowledge of the student." She encourages recommendation-letter writers to "embrace the task" and approach it as a "creative journey," with capturing the "essence" of the student, resident, or fellow or colleague up for promotion as the goal (6). Selecting adjectives and attributes to describe the person you are recommending are a key part of the process. To do this, Whalley encourages visualization of the person being recommended now, and in the future, with an eye to the qualities that will make them successful.

Specific Advice for Writing Recommendation Letters

Never agree to write a recommendation letter for someone you do not believe should get the position or award you would be recommending for. This is a waste of valuable time and a disservice to both the person you are recommending without enthusiasm and the company, hospital, or graduate school to which the letter is going. If vindictiveness is driving you to write the letter, put this emotion away—it will only backfire. Rather, let the requestor know that you are unable to write the "glowing" or "excellent" letter you know he or she would like to see and gently suggest that he or she seek a recommendation letter elsewhere. It is not your business after this. You will be rid of the painful and potentially dishonest chore of recommending someone you feel is not fit for the position or the award. If the person asks you to explain why you cannot recommend him or her, you do not need to honestly say what your reservations are but only that you do not feel comfortable writing the "excellent" recommendation that he or she may deserve. Usually students, residents, fellows, and peers take the hint and move to greener pastures for the recommendation letter.

In my recommendation letters, the first sentence says, "I am delighted to recommend _____ [full name] for _____ [position, scholarship, graduate school, etc.] at _____." The next sentence indicates in what capacity you know the student, resident, fellow, or faculty member. Indicate for how long you have known the person. You may be or have been his or her advisor, tutor, mentor, colleague, collaborator, fellow committee member, or co-teacher. You may have known the person for three months or twelve years.

If the organization the person is being recommended to requires that you note what the person's standing in your organization is, the third sentence will state, "_____ [full name] is a [student, resident, fellow, or faculty member] in excellent standing at _____ [the particular medical school, hospital program or hospital]."

Include in the first paragraph major high school honors, awards, and leadership experience. Note if he or she was valedictorian or salutatorian for the high school, as well as the number of students in the graduating class.

I ask each of the fourth-year students whose dean's letter I am writing to check with his or her family about their high school honors, such as National Merit Scholarship winner or semifinalist or finalist for the National Merit Scholarship or having received a Letter of Commendation from the National Merit Scholarship Corporation, as a way of recognizing the student's superior standardized test–taking abilities. Noting that the student was an advanced placement scholar is a similarly useful as a way of confirming his or her standardized test–taking abilities. Include major scholarships to college, particularly if they were for all four years, and significant athletic awards and leadership in athletics, such as being the captain of the track and field team that won the state championship that year. Musical prowess is also touted, particularly if the student was in an orchestra and played first violin, first flute, etc.

For college awards, give the degree earned, the field in which it was earned, the year, and whether it was with honors or distinction. Also note the college grade-point average if it was outstanding, and give the years the student made the dean's list. Include scholarships won while in college. List the major graduation honors. Summarize key research experiences, the mentor who supervised the person's research, and the funding for the project. Detail any community service, teaching, tutoring, or leadership activities. If the person has extracurricular activities (such as singing in a chorus or volunteering at a homeless shelter), describe this and note if he or she founded the volunteer activity or had a major leadership role, such as being the manager for the orchestra, in charge of a budget of $50,000 per year.

For graduating medical school students, discuss their awards and honors, research work, community service, leadership, and teaching activities. Note the sources of project funding, scholarships won, and summer research grants. Showcase full-year research grants from the Howard Hughes Medical Institute, the Doris Duke Foundation, and the Cloister Program at NIH. Comment on other degrees that have been completed or are near completion, such as the master of public health, master of public policy, or master of business administration. Recognize laboratory or epidemiological research and name the mentor. Note if any presentation or publication has resulted from the research work. Discuss teaching experience with medical students as a tutor or a leader in a preclinical or clinical teaching activity or innovation. Note foreign language competency and fluency by saying, "This person is fluent in conversational Spanish and competent in medical Spanish." If the student has been active in the annual Broadway-style spoof of the faculty, the Medical School Olympics, or athletic competitions, note these activities under extracurricular activities.

In the next paragraph, include quotes from the comments of the first- and second-year tutors if the person is a medical or dental student. These quotes indicate the student's level of preparation and participation in the preclinical years. Select required clinical evaluations from the third- and fourth-year clerkships, quoting the entire summative comments verbatim. If you are recommending a resident or fellow, you will not likely have access to the comments from other faculty, unless you are the residency director. Describe your interactions with the resident or fellow, his or her clinical acumen, bedside manner, and politeness to the patients and their families. Comment on record-keeping abilities and conscientiousness in following up on patients' problems, laboratory and radiologic results, and on the ability to write focused but complete progress notes.

At the end of the letter, crystallize in a few well-constructed sentences the unique and wonderful personal qualities of the student, resident, fellow, or faculty member. Summarize the major accomplishments in a paragraph that places the person's defining qualities and top achievements into high relief. Write a final sentence indicating the estimated future trajectory for the student, resident, fellow, or faculty member in glowing and optimistic terms. Note that you are glad to give your "highest recommendation" to this person, "without reservations."

For a faculty promotion, focus on the person's teaching excellence; in your position as a medical teacher, you are usually asked to recommend a faculty member because he or she has taught in a course that you are directing or leading. This faculty member has indicated that teaching expertise is an important component of the promotion package. Use verbatim any excellent comments that were made in the evaluations for the course or the teaching exercise. This gives a valid ring to your claim in the letter that this person is an excellent teacher.

✶ TEACHING TIPS

1. Align your test questions with your teaching objectives; examinations should not be unpleasant surprises.
2. Familiarize yourself with what the National Board of Medical Examiners is expecting students and residents to know in your specialty area; make sure your teaching covers this material.
3. Save all old exam questions; they are your make-up exams.
4. Audience-response systems increase class participation and enthusiasm for learning; the jury is still out on whether they improve understanding and retention.
5. Prepare for the OSCE with specific teaching points and visual aids to supplement the learning; stay on time and finish evaluations promptly.
6. Make evaluations easier by obtaining a copy of the form you are expected to fill out so that you can be looking for the required skills, knowledge, attitudes, and behaviors as you are working with the person to be evaluated.
7. Have a template for letters that you consistently use; the more letters of recommendation you write, the better and faster you become.

✶ TAKE-HOME POINTS

- Be an ally, not a foe, in all areas of assessment.
- Making up good tests is hard to do; learn how.

- A failing grade is worth looking at again; develop a plan for the student to succeed via remediation.
- Set yourself up for easy rather than difficult feedback sessions; use "chapter and verse" from your own observations to guide what you say.
- Writing great letters of recommendation requires dedicated time and a foolproof system; develop both to avoid disappointing applicants who trust you to complete this important activity by the deadline.
- If you enjoy praising another person's numerous accomplishments, recommendation letters are fun to do.

CHAPTER SEVEN

Preclinical Teaching

- 🦋 *How do I run a preclinical course successfully?*
- 🦋 *What is problem-based learning, and why should I use it?*
- 🦋 *How do I write a problem-based learning case?*
- 🦋 *What constitutes faculty development for preclinical tutors?*
- 🦋 *How can I be a successful tutor in a preclinical science course?*
- 🦋 *What keeps a small group engaged in learning science?*
- 🦋 *What do students want from a lecturer?*

Effective Organization of a Preclinical Course

Students and teachers frequently laugh during and at the end of the gastrointestinal pathophysiology course that I direct. Granted, this is the last course of the second year. It immediately precedes Step 1 of the USMLE and the students' entrance into their primary clinical clerkship year. But that's not why they laugh. They laugh because students know from the rumor mill and from firsthand experience that the course is well run, well taught, and packed with information they need to know for the boards and the wards. They can relax and sit back while my well-trained team and I roll out a dazzling intellectual feast. It will be fun, productive, and stimulating—no waste of their time when they are stressed about boards. They can afford to laugh in the tutorials, the small groups, and the pathology laboratories. Students are highly regarded and well taken care of in the gastrointestinal pathophysiology block. Too often, course directors behave in an adversarial manner toward students. A negative, adversarial, or sarcastic attitude will get you nowhere with bright, but beleaguered, medical students.

My tip is to construct your preclinical course with *LAFS* (pronounced "laughs") so that you also have students and teachers laughing in a fun and pleasant way. What is *LAFS*?

L stands for following a *logical order*. In the gastrointestinal pathophysiology course, a logical order means presenting organs in a logical sequence, starting with the mouth (beginning with the tongue as an important muscular organ in the process of swallowing), then going to the esophagus, stomach,

- Seven organs taught in the following sequence:
  - Week 1: Esophagus, Stomach, Duodenum
  - Week 2: Small and Large Intestine, Pancreas
  - Week 3: Liver, Gall Bladder, Biliary Tract

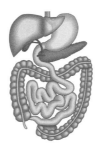

Figure 7.1. **Logical Progressions and Integration**
Demonstrate a logical pathway in the ordering of course, elective, lecture, small-group, or tutorial material. Weave the content into a cohesive, integrated whole using segues and links to appropriate material.

duodenum, small and large bowels, pancreas, biliary tract, and liver (fig. 7.1). The course covers these organs in two and a half weeks, with four days per week allotted to pathophysiology. My official teaching time for each of the ten days of the course runs for four and a half hours, from 8 a.m. to 12:30 p.m. Educational sessions may be scheduled after 12:30 p.m., but these are classified as optional on the course calendar. Even though each session is taped for students to watch, material found only in these optional sessions would not be on our final exam or midcourse quiz, but it could be on the Step 1, USMLE, and will be seen on the wards. We highlight these content areas for this reason.

Why is a logical order so important? I know what an illogical order does to students' opinion of medical school teaching, because the very first course that I helped run at Harvard Medical School in 1993 used an illogical order. This course received the worst teaching evaluations I have ever seen. Needless to say, when I was asked to be the director of the gastrointestinal pathophysiology course in 1994, I never looked back at an illogical order, but started from scratch to create a logically ordered course that would be given accolades rather than boos.

A means *approaching* the same topic from multiple, overlapping *angles* (fig. 7.2). An example from the gastrointestinal pathophysiology course follows: On the first day of the course, the lower esophageal sphincter is discussed in tutorial (8–9:30 a.m.). Multiple diagrams are provided of the innervation of the sphincter, the anatomy of the diaphragm in relationship to the sphincter, the multiple reasons why gastroesophageal reflux may occur, and the consequences of low sphincter pressure. The tutor shows color photographs of the endoscopic appearance of the distal esophagus, both normal and abnormal, as well as photomicrographs of Barrett's epithelium with and without low-grade dysplasia on a plasma screen in the tutorial room. The problem-based tutorial case focuses on an obese man named Louis Garrison, who has severe

A. Multiple Teaching Venues

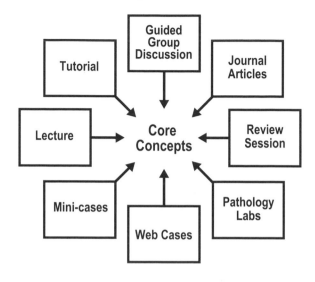

B. Teaching the Pathophysiology of Jaundice

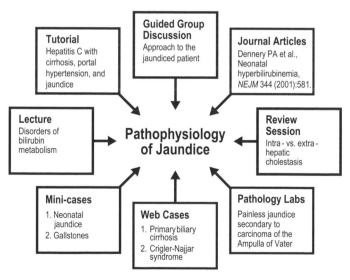

Figure 7.2. **Teaching the Same Topic from Multiple Overlapping Angles**
Use a variety of teaching venues to expose the students, residents, fellows, or peer group to the same topic in multiple ways and from multiple angles. This method gives ample opportunity for comprehension of even the most complex topic.

reflux and Barrett's esophagus. Following the tutorial, students hear a lecture on the esophagus in which the importance of adequate contractile pressure in the lower esophageal sphincter is explained along with its innervation, relationship to the crural diaphragm, and the many reasons why reflux can occur. Barrett's esophagus is discussed as one of the major complications of gastroesophageal reflux. The students then break out into small groups for ninety minutes (11 a.m.–12:30 p.m.) for a mini-case session, which is an interactive question-and-answer session with one teacher for fifteen to twenty-five students (depending on the room sizes available at the medical school for the class of approximately one hundred seventy students).

The mini-case session for the esophagus focuses on the yin/yang of high pressure versus low pressure of the lower esophageal sphincter and the clinical correlates of each. Each group reviews a case of dysphagia due to achalasia, with chest x-rays showing the widened mediastinum caused by a giant dilated esophagus, a bird's beak on a barium swallow, classic manometric findings of aperistalsis, elevated lower esophageal sphincter pressure with failure to relax to baseline gastric pressure with swallowing, diagrams of the pathophysiology, followed by diagrams detailing the pathophysiologic reasoning behind the multiple treatment options. The achalasia case (yin) is paired with a case of scleroderma (yang) in which a markedly low pressure in the lower esophageal sphincter, secondary to atrophy, and fibrosis of lower esophageal muscles, due to ischemic damage, is the pathophysiologic concept, while severe reflux, nighttime coughing, and an esophageal stricture are key clinical presentations. Visual aids include an abnormal barium upper gastrointestinal series showing a stricture of the distal esophagus in a patient who has classic features of scleroderma, such as sclerodactly, facial telangiectasias, Raynaud syndrome, resulting in blanching of the fingertips in the cold, sclerodactly, and Barrett's epithelium on endoscopic biopsy.

The review session the following day highlights the differential diagnosis for dysphagia, the innervation of the esophagus, the mechanisms for the high-pressure zone of the lower esophageal sphincter, what factors elevate lower esophageal sphincter pressure, and what factors decrease it in patients who have reflux esophagitis or scleroderma. That same day, a pediatric abdominal surgeon reviews the anatomy of the gastrointestinal tract in a lecture. He shows a video clip of a laparoscopic Heller's myotomy performed on a child who has achalasia. Three days later, the upper gastrointestinal pathology laboratory discusses a case of Barrett's esophagus and its progression to dysplasia and adenocarcinoma. The students watch three video clips of upper endoscopy footage during the pathology laboratory, showing a normal esophagus, Barrett's esophagus, and adenocarcinoma of the esophagus.

There are quiz questions at the end of the first full week of class related to the lower esophageal sphincter as well as questions in the pathology quiz at the beginning of the pathology laboratory. During the final three-hour review session, one hour is spent reviewing the pathophysiology of the esophagus and stomach, so that students' misconceptions can be cleared up one last time before the final exam in the course and before they take Step 1 of the USMLE. The Harvard Medical School aggregate score for the Step 1 section on gastrointestinal diseases has been excellent in the past few years, with the majority of the students' scores well above the national average.

I find teaching the same pathophysiologic concept from multiple different, but overlapping, angles leads to better understanding and retention of the material. Students greatly appreciate repetition. The different ways of viewing the same concept of the lower esophageal sphincter, from colorful artist's renditions to endoscopic videos, to having them draw the lower esophageal sphincter on the blackboard in tutorial, diagramming how a hiatal hernia alters the relationship of the bolstering effect of the diaphragm on the sphincter, is extremely helpful. Their learning is further increased by exposure to the different manometric and x-ray patterns for the high- (achalasia) versus low-pressure (scleroderma) illnesses. Layering similar material and coming at the same concept from different angles helps the students to gain confidence that they understand a moderately complicated pathophysiologic concept. When we arrive at a complicated concept such as portal hypertension, with increased resistance in the liver from fibrosis and high flow in the portal system from splanchnic vasodilatation, we use the same overlapping principle, coming from multiple angles at portal hypertension with tutorial diagrams, videos of esophageal variceal banding, pathology laboratory photomicrographs of different types of cirrhosis, lecture slides, algorithms, lecture notes, and required references on stellate cells, and on the proposed mechanisms for portal hypertension. In addition, we have an hour-long review session to reinforce the students' understanding of why portal hypertension occurs and what factors sustain it.

F is for the *formula* for successful teaching of any topic in preclinical medical education. I have developed this formula through fifteen years of trial and error as course director for Harvard Medical School's second-year course on gastrointestinal pathophysiology. The formula consists of two *E*'s and two *R*'s: *exposition, exploration, reiteration,* and *review* (table 7.1).

Let's look at what these words mean. *Exposition* simply means showing or using a patient case, anecdote, or vignette to anchor the student's interest in the underlying pathophysiologic process. The exposition of clinical material gets the student hooked on wanting to understand pathophysiology and creates a better chance that he or she may remember the concepts because of the reality of the case material. The popularity and effectiveness of using a case or a vignette stems from recognizing the needs of adult learners. As noted in the section on adult learning theory in chapter 5, adults approach learning as a problem-solving exercise. Adults enjoy and learn when participants with different expertise and backgrounds work on a realistic problem in small groups, as occurs in a problem-based tutorial or in a larger-group case-based learning session.

Exploration refers to students' having the opportunity in class, tutorial sessions, small groups, or pathology laboratories to talk to their fellow students about understanding the key points or objectives of the case. Usually a faculty member guides the discussion, but some course directors prefer tutorless tutorials or problem-set sessions in which students work with other students to examine the material, its implications, and the concepts it is showcasing. Exploration relies primarily on asking questions and covering objectives. Tutors as well as pathologists and mini-case leaders ask questions and cover objectives. Time is given in tutorial and pathology labs for the students to talk to each other and help each other understand concepts. In the small-group sessions, the students answer prepared questions they can look up the answers to beforehand and share with the group. Students, as well as the teacher, do the teaching in these sessions. In the focused discussion sessions, in which the material is particularly complex, less student-to-student teaching is done, but

Table 7.1. Educational Formula for Course Organization

Exposition of concepts in lecture, focused discussion, and mini-cases

Exploration in tutorials, small-group sessions, and laboratories

Reiteration of concepts in other types of teaching exercises and required readings

Review of concepts in an end-of-week session

the teacher explores the pathophysiology as a running monologue with slides and diagrams. Students jump in with their own questions, which stimulate further explanations from the teacher.

Questions as the Ultimate Teaching Tool

Questions are the best teaching tool to engage an audience, whether the audience is elementary school children, business school students, or medical school students. Audiences want to participate and to use their collective wisdom. The audience-response systems have made this point amply clear. Audiences want to actively engage, share, be put on the spot, and have their opinions heard rather than be passive. Adult-learner audiences do not mind being wrong; they see questions and answers as a way to learn.

Questions encourage preparation for the teaching session if they are given out beforehand. They make it possible for everyone to participate if the discussion leader is skilled at eliciting responses from the quiet student, resident, or peer. Make your questions crystal clear, concise, and open-ended for discussion. Discussion questions should not have a simple fill-in-the-blank right answer; ideally, they are open to as many interpretations as there are participants. Questions should probe the reasoning behind the answer so that logic, familiarity with content, and synthesis are demonstrated. Using guiding questions in tutorial has transformed our gastrointestinal preclinical pathophysiology tutorial into a dynamic, vibrant learning environment that showcases each student's preparation and participation readily and permits the tutor (discussion leader) to actively, but gently, guide and steer the discussion to fruitful coverage of the learning objectives for each tutorial session.

R is for *reiteration.* I am not ashamed to say the same thing twice. Medical students, even the best and brightest, appreciate your explaining complex concepts more than once. Thus, pathology laboratories follow the pathology lectures, reiterating what was said in lecture, but using different examples and adding clinical vignettes, x-rays, endoscopic photos, videos, and surgical findings. The pathology quiz that begins each pathology laboratory takes its images from the lecture that preceded it, reiterating the image as important to remember. Rather than being annoyed by the duplication, students compliment us on this mode of getting the important images and facts to stick in their heads. Students want faculty or course directors to separate the wheat from the chaff, the priority items from the trivial, and the knowledge that is likely to be on the boards or their ward rotations from the fly-by-night items that will rarely be seen again. It is incumbent on course directors to think long and hard about the facts, concepts, and morphology that are reiterated because the students need to know and understand these bottom-line "take-aways."

R is for *review*. Review is not the same educational tool as reiteration. Review means establishing formal review sessions on a weekly basis, specifically to go over, in moderate depth, the concepts rather than the clinical facts. Clinical facts, such as norovirus being found in outbreaks of diarrhea on cruise ships, and turtles and pet iguanas being carriers of *Salmonella*, inevitably creep into review sessions to lighten the session. Review also applies to having weekly quizzes that are self-graded or counted for credit, and prepathology self-assessment quizzes to let students see how well they understood or grasped the lecture material immediately before the laboratory begins. Review does not mean regurgitate. The material chosen for a review session is carefully screened. It has been stripped to its barest bones so that the students who are confused can finally get the concept straight. All final exam material *must* appear in a review session in one form or other, or the students will not deem the review sessions important. Next year's class will not attend the review sessions in full force, given the lack of a relationship between what you teach in the review and what you consider essential to test. Your review sessions and your tests should be completely aligned if you wish the review sessions to draw the desired crowd of interested students. Review sessions are a last opportunity to make up for some less-than-ideal small-group session leaders, tutors, or pathology laboratory instructors. Try to deliver a cogent, clear, enthusiastic, and engaging review of the high points of your course in a videotaped review session, which can be viewed by the students who do not come at a later time.

S stands for having a *system*. A preclinical course requires a reliable and responsive system for smoothly, efficiently, and quietly making the teaching happen with the least fuss and angst for both teachers and students. Harvard Medical School and Harvard Business School have whole departments devoted to smoothing out the mechanics of teaching for students and teachers. Course organization includes producing the course calendars and syllabi, recruiting teachers, creating the lists of students for tutorials, laboratories, and small groups, and scheduling rooms, organizing faculty meetings, and assessing audiovisual requirements. These tasks are performed by skilled administrators who enjoy interacting with students and faculty. In the gastrointestinal pathophysiology course, almost eighty teachers are used for the two-and-a-half-week course due to the numerous small-group sessions. The best course in the world is only as good as its weakest administrator. Hours of work by faculty can go down the drain if the wrong answer key is posted, the wrong quiz is given, the rooms are not reserved, the students are not properly distributed, and the syllabus is missing key objectives or required readings. I have been fortunate to have the same wonderful head course manager for more than six years and the same outstanding executive director of curriculum support. The course manager's assistant has been a huge help with photocopying, syllabus production, putting together teacher packets for faculty guides and references, and stocking faculty lockers with reference books and course materials. I insist on an organized and painless course for students and faculty, but this requires great energy and commitment on the part of the course manager, her assistant, and me and my teaching fellow. Each student complaint is taken seriously, especially when it involves an organizational glitch or recommended syllabus improvement. These types of complaint are generally readily fixable. Once we have fixed the problem, we will alert the entire class to the solution.

An important part of the system has been having a teaching fellow for the course. Each year the teaching fellow works alongside me for the several months beforehand. We rehearse, rehash, and redesign the course in the weeks before the course, during the course, and after the course is over. During the course, the fellow is both tutor and a small-group leader for all sessions. He or she gives part of the weekly review sessions. He or she is my confidant, constant companion, and valuable and independent set of eyes and ears during the course. We sit together during all lectures and special sessions. Our roles are rehearsed before each presentation. Each recent fellow has also participated in an educational research project as an outgrowth of the course. This work has resulted in their being a co-author on an educational publication.

Implementing *LAFS* may be done as a multistep process over several years, as I have done with my course. First, I changed the logic of how the organs were presented. I carefully thought out the position of bile salts. An understanding of bile salts is required to understand fat absorption when we are talking about the small intestine (second week), as well as for the formation of gallstones, when we are talking about the liver (third week). Second, I decided on the course objectives, focusing on which concepts and diseases should receive the most time. Third, once I had decided on the objectives, I designed a course schedule that would allow me to teach important concepts from different angles in different types of educational sessions. This layered course schedule provides multiple opportunities for students to comprehend concepts.

Using the formula of exposition, exploration, reiteration, and review permits the teacher to write memorable cases, which lead to questions and curiosity on the part of the students. Reiterating important points more than once sets the stage for the students acquiring an active and important body of knowledge that is essential for the boards and wards. Reviewing in a lecture hall–style venue all exam material and all key concepts before the final exam creates good will among the students toward the course and its faculty.

Problem-based Learning

Although problem-based learning has not been shown to increase standardized test scores, it is an enjoyable method of small-group learning. Medical education literature supports problem-based learning as having the following positive benefits:

- Aids in the successful retrieval of information
- Helps develop problem-solving skills
- Promotes critical thinking
- Fosters interpersonal communication and team-building skills
- Encourages the skills needed for life-long learning

Problem-based learning has become a prominent and popular method of teaching in medical school partly for the reasons listed above (Armstrong 1991; Barrows and Tamblyn 1980; Barrows 1988; Tosteson, Adelstein, and Carver 1994; Wetzel 1994). A real-life case concerning real-life medical dilemmas encourages the remembrance and retrieval of the medical and scientific concepts associated with understanding the case and the answers to the questions the case raises. The traditional problem-based learning methodology involves the evaluation of a problem by the participants in a small-group setting with a facilitator. There are three major components to the active learning that occurs in a problem-based session: (1) the participants identify the facts presented in the case, (2) the participants generate hypotheses based on these facts, and (3) the participants identify the learning issues that need to be researched or studied. In a problem-based session, the participants typically drive the learning. They work together to solve the problem. Cases are real-life situations and unfold realistically to simulate the interactions between patient and physician and the decision-making process that occurs. Multidisciplinary learning is fostered. The teacher acts as a facilitator, who probes the reasoning process, provides feedback, prevents dominance by a single participant or a few participants, and prevents major digressions. Although the learning objectives for the case underlie the problem set forth in the case, they are traditionally not known at the outset to the participants but are discovered as the case unfolds.

Significant teacher preparation and training are essential to the smooth running of each session. However, the rewards for the teacher and participants are vibrant and memorable discussions about real-life medical and scientific problems that solidify knowledge and the understanding of key concepts. A recent study noted that problem-based learning had positive effects on physician competencies, particularly in the appreciation of the social and emotional aspects of health care and in self-directed learning (Koh et al. 2008).

Integrating Business School Teaching Strategies into Pathophysiology Tutorials

Taylor and Miflin (2008) pointed out the enormous variability in problem-based learning at different medical schools and even within the same medical school. We recently changed the role of the tutor in a problem-based tutorial to a discussion leader (Christensen 1991a, 1991b). In the following paragraphs, I outline some of the educational principles that have guided me (Shields et al. 2007). I hope they will be helpful to others who are organizing the teaching of pathophysiology to preclinical medical and dental students.

Nine years ago, I received a grant from Harvard Medical School to change the role of the tutor from a facilitator to a discussion leader, who uses questions and summaries to be a more active participant in the discussion of pathophysiology. Our methods for faculty development were based on the discussion-teaching model used at the Harvard Business School and Harvard's Kennedy School of Government (Christensen 1991a, 1991b). Although the gastrointestinal pathophysiology course had always been popular, the faculty development changes have significantly improved the course ratings.

Traditional problem-based learning has been participant centered, and the facilitator has been encouraged to be an active listener rather than a discussion leader. Recently, at Harvard Medical School, we changed the problem-based teaching style in the gastrointestinal pathophysiology course for second-year students to reflect the discussion-leadership strategies that have been successful in promoting active learning in graduate schools of business, government, and education (Shields et al. 2007). The gastrointestinal faculty made these changes to increase the engagement of the students in the small-group tutorials, improve the students' preparation and participation in the discussion, and enhance the vibrancy and quality of the discussion. Specifically, we changed tutor's role from that of a passive facilitator to that of an active discussion leader, who asks questions to encourage discussion and understanding of the educational objectives. In addition, we added three new structural elements: (1) a pretutorial announcement of the key objectives to be covered during each session and the distribution of the pertinent pages of the case beforehand, (2) an end-of-tutorial summary given by the tutor, and (3) a visual map of the major points of the discussion in the form of a closure schematic or colorful "placemat." Giving out the objectives beforehand has encouraged preparation, while the end-of-tutorial summary and closure schematic have reinforced the important learning objectives of the discussion and clarified concepts. Our alterations been have widely applauded by both students and faculty, who have commented on the increased transmission of knowledge and understanding of concepts during the tutorial.

To develop cases for problem-based learning sessions, identify the objectives that form the basis for the case's development. What scientific or medical points or concepts do you wish to teach? How do you get them across with a particular case? Who is the audience? How much time do you have? What are some of the great clinical cases that are relevant to the science you are trying to explain?

Keep a record of all great x-rays, pathology and endoscopic photographs, and EKGs from your clinical cases, with a notation of the patient's medical record number, so that this unique material is available for your educational purposes.

Steps to Making Sessions Problem Free

1. Define the learning objectives for each individual session.
2. Determine audience, size of group, site of discussion, time frame, and level of prior knowledge.
3. Design a clinical case from real-life patients to stimulate discussion of the learning objectives.
4. Train faculty in content areas, the use of visual aids, discussion leadership, group dynamics, and the art of summarization.
5. Test the problem-based learning case on a pilot group and make adjustments accordingly.

6. Use the case with the intended audience and have the discussion leader ask both predetermined and spontaneously generated questions to help direct the flow of the discussion effectively.

7. Obtain feedback from participants and faculty on the strengths and weaknesses of the case and the questions that were asked to accomplish the learning objectives.

8. Revise the case to stimulate an active and vibrant discussion that increases the participants' knowledge and their interest in pursuing further learning in the area.

Steps to Writing a Case

1. The teacher or course director identifies the relevant basic science or clinical medicine concepts to be discussed. These become the objectives for the case and form the basis for the development of the case. The learning objectives drive the teacher's preparation and the student's learning agenda and their mutual discussion.

2. The teacher or course director chooses an appropriate case. The case should stimulate curiosity, interest, and questions. It should encourage the formation of hypotheses. The case is written about a patient with one main problem and contains the information needed to discuss and attempt to solve the issues that the case raises. The problem in the case is concretely formulated, has a degree of complexity, and should be commonly seen in medical practice. Problems usually represent urgent or life-threatening situations and have potentially serious outcomes. Prevention or therapeutic intervention can make a significant difference in prognosis. There are multiple possible case formats. Paper cases may be descriptive and unfold over two or three separate sessions, or they may be a short story used in one session. Cases may be vignettes or mini-cases, with only one brief paragraph and one main focus of disease, or may be only a bulleted item, with one or two sentences.

3. The teacher or course director begins writing the case by mentally reviewing patients he or she has seen with an illness or dilemma that underlies the educational goals and objectives. The writer should begin with the questions: Who is the audience? What is my teaching goal? The story should be written as if telling it to a person who is

not a physician. Several patients' histories, physical exams, and laboratory data may be meshed to create the case.

4. The case should be developed from a real-life situation and not be a contrived or "classic" textbook description. The case should serve one purpose. It should contain accurate data. Information should be added or deleted to keep focus on the main goal.

5. The case should be critically evaluated as a teaching tool by piloting it in a small session with interested reviewers.

Steps to Implementing the Case

1. Identify the audience who would benefit most from the learning objectives of the case (i.e., students, residents, attending faculty, nurses).

2. Identify the group size. Is it a group of five, ten, fifteen, twenty-five, or fifty participants? What is the venue: a tutorial room, a classroom, or an amphitheatre-style classroom?

3. Determine the expected time frame for the case discussion. Is it thirty, sixty, or ninety minutes?

4. Photocopy the description of the case and collate it page by page for ease of distribution to the group.

5. Include a list of objectives, a bibliography, and a description of the teaching aids, such as x-rays, pathology, and endoscopic photographs, on a separate sheet.

Steps to Effective Case Writing

Hafler (1989) clearly outlines the steps to take to effective cases.

1. Define the basic science or clinical medicine concepts to be taught.

2. Create learning objectives.

3. Answer the following questions: Who is the audience? What are the teaching goals? What is the time frame?

4. Use a clinical scenario that illustrates the concepts to be learned.

5. Formula for a good case for discussion:
   - Depicts a common, potentially serious or life-threatening problem.
   - Contains an element of mystery.
   - Builds momentum.

- Generates controversy.
- Is supported by excellent visuals.

6. Choose an appropriate case from your files. It may be a composite.
    - Use real-life situations.
    - Have the case unfold realistically, usually over the course of two or three sessions.
    - The problem should encourage decision making.

A Harvard Medical School Example

Harvard Medical School's gastrointestinal pathophysiology course offers a good example of a problem-based learning case on colon cancer and colon polyp genetics. The case has the following objectives:

1. Understand the importance of the family history in the development of colonic adenomas and colon cancer.
2. Diagram the adenoma to carcinoma sequence. Note the specific role of the APC, K-ras, P53, and SMAD 4 genes. Define an adenoma and compare it to a hyperplastic polyp.
3. Distinguish tubular from villous adenoma and explain the prognostic differences between the two types.
4. Recognize the different types of polyp found in Peutz-Jeghers syndrome, juvenile polyposis syndrome, and familial adenomatous polyposis.
5. Discuss the genetic abnormalities that underlie familial adenomatous polyposis, attenuated familial adenomatous polyposis, MYH-associated polyposis, and hereditary nonpolyposis colon cancer.
6. Recognize the extra-colonic malignancies that are associated with hereditary nonpolyposis colon cancer.
7. Define the difference between synchronous and metachronous colon cancer and distinguish the risk for occurrence of synchronous and metachronous lesions in sporadic colon cancer versus hereditary nonpolyposis colon cancer syndrome.
8. Describe the rationale behind the use of aspirin or NSAIDs to decrease the risk of colon cancer and the recurrence of adenomatous polyps.
9. Explain the pros and cons of colonoscopy compared to virtual colonoscopy for the identification of polyps and cancers for the average-risk patient and the high-risk patient.

The case concerns a 64-year-old management consultant who complains to his primary care physician about blood in his stool for the past six months. On rectal exam, his physician notes that his prostate is enlarged and his stool negative for occult blood. There is a family history of colon cancer in his uncle, at age 52, and colon polyps are present in his younger brother, age 57. His two sisters are well. He does not know what type of polyp his brother had removed, but his brother has a colonoscopy every few years. He had himself been told to have a colonoscopy several years ago, but when he heard that the procedure was uncomfortable and the preparation for it was drinking a gallon of bad-tasting solution, he decided not to have it done.

The primary care physician refers him to a gastroenterologist who finds two polyps in the colon, but the quality of preparation is poor and the patient is asked to return in one year rather than the every-three-year interval recommended because of his family history. The pathology report indicates that the two polyps are adenomas. The patient is asked to obtain his brother's reports. His brother's polyps are adenomas. The patient is placed on aspirin as possible chemoprevention for colon cancer, although he is warned about the possibility of gastrointestinal bleeding secondary to the aspirin.

One year later, the patient undergoes a colonoscopy and three more adenomas are found, one of which is 2 cm in size, is villous and sessile in appearance, and is located in the ascending colon. The endoscopist removes the lesion in pieces. The pathology shows adenomatous tissue with high-grade dysplasia, and the patient is brought back one month later for follow-up. A small amount of polyp regrowth is noted at the same spot and shows high-grade dysplasia. The patient is referred for a right colectomy. A focus of invasive cancer is found in the specimen. The cancer is TNM stage $T_2 N_0 M_0$.

Since then, three more years have passed. Only two adenomas of less than 0.5 cm have been noted on the yearly colonoscopies. The patient asks if he can have a virtual colonoscopy instead. He notes that one sister has developed uterine cancer and the other ovarian cancer. He is referred for genetic testing.

This sixty-minute case generates many excellent questions and is used as a springboard for the faculty expert's discussion of colon cancer genetics.

Faculty Development for Tutors

Faculty members require training in both content and concepts as well as in the skills of facilitation and discussion leadership (Steinert et al. 2006; Tavakol, Dennick, and Tavakol 2009). Specifically, faculty should be trained in:

1. Using questions to further discussion along productive lines
2. Engaging the quiet student and modulating the dominant student
3. Summarizing the discussion at the end
4. Discussing a closure schematic or colorful 11 x 17 inch "placemat" at the time of the summary to clarify concepts and reiterate important take-home points

Faculty should be provided with key references, book chapters, and a specific weekly teaching session emphasizing content to maximize their ability to question, listen, and respond and to summarize the discussion.

New tutors attend three faculty development sessions. The first session (two hours and forty-five minutes) is devoted to learning how to ask various types of question, modulate student dynamics, and summarize the ninety-minute discussion. The necessity of functioning as a discussion leader who guides the discussion to cover the pertinent objectives requires that the tutor ask questions to stimulate discussion or to steer discussion toward topics that might otherwise not be covered. A mock tutorial that uses questions to move the discussion in different directions is part of the teaching session. Tutors are also shown videos of quiet and dominant students to help them enunciate their options for managing tutorial dynamics by bringing in the quiet student, modulating the dominant student, and fostering an environment that encourages mutual respect and participation. A faculty expert demonstrates the art of summarizing with a case discussion and a mock class in which participants attempt to make a decision on a controversial topic. The faculty expert summarizes the class discussion and conclusions.

The second two and one-half hour session focuses on expert knowledge, summaries, and closure schematics, as well as the integration of cross-cultural care into the tutorial, with the use of specific case triggers. See the section in chapter 10 entitled "Cross-Cultural Care," describing this part of the faculty development program in detail. The course director reviews pathophysiologic concepts for the upcoming cases. Tutors are taught to summarize the ninety-minute tutorial in three to five minutes, using a closure schematic, or "placemat," that visually outlines the important concepts (fig. 7.3). Each student will be given a handout of the schematic to follow the tutor as he or she emphasizes the important take-home points and mechanisms. The evaluation form to measure a tutor's teaching capabilities is shown to the tutors so that each sees the criteria by which he or she will be judged. A study focusing on

Gastroesophageal Reflux

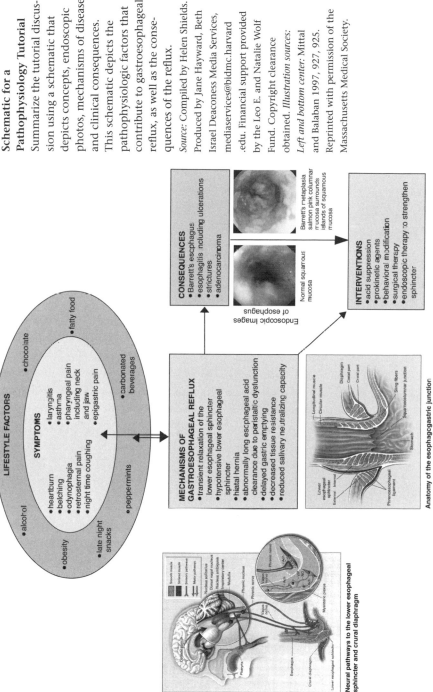

Figure 7.3. **Summary Schematic for a Pathophysiology Tutorial**

Summarize the tutorial discussion using a schematic that depicts concepts, endoscopic photos, mechanisms of disease, and clinical consequences. This schematic depicts the pathophysiologic factors that contribute to gastroesophageal reflux, as well as the consequences of the reflux.

Source: Compiled by Helen Shields. Produced by Jane Hayward, Beth Israel Deaconess Media Services, mediaservices@bidmc.harvard.edu. Financial support provided by the Leo E. and Natalie Wolf Fund. Copyright clearance obtained. *Illustration sources: Left and bottom center:* Mittal and Balaban 1997, 927, 925. Reprinted with permission of the Massachusetts Medical Society.

LIFESTYLE FACTORS

- alcohol
- obesity
- late night snacks
- peppermints
- carbonated beverages
- chocolate
- fatty food

SYMPTOMS

- heartburn
- belching
- odynophagia
- retrosternal pain
- night time coughing
- laryngitis
- asthma
- pharyngeal pain including neck and jaw
- epigastric pain

MECHANISMS OF GASTROESOPHAGEAL REFLUX

- transient relaxation of the lower esophageal sphincter
- hypotensive lower esophageal sphincter
- hiatal hernia
- abnormally long esophageal acid clearance due to peristaltic dysfunction
- delayed gastric emptying
- decreased tissue resistance
- reduced salivary neutralizing capacity

Anatomy of the esophagogastric junction

CONSEQUENCES

- Barrett's esophagus
- esophagitis including ulcerations
- strictures
- adenocarcinoma

Endoscopic Images of esophagus

Normal squamous mucosa

Barrett's metaplasia salmon pink columnar mucosa surrounds islands of squamous mucosa

INTERVENTIONS

- acid suppression
- prokinetic agents
- behavioral modification
- surgical therapy
- endoscopic therapy to strengthen sphincter

Neural pathways to the lower esophageal sphincter and crural diaphragm when the tutor decides to intervene in a problem-based tutorial showed how complex the decision can be (Lee et al. 2009).

The third session is one hour long, meets in a tutorial room, and is primarily directed toward new tutors, yet the majority of experienced tutors come to refresh their memories about the specific details of the course. This session focuses on the mechanics of running a tutorial group, including available written materials, Web resources, visual aids in the form of endoscopic and pathologic images, and locker location and combination. The importance of individual meetings, with the seven to nine tutorial students for feedback sessions regarding the student's preparation and participation in tutorial, is emphasized, along with specific instructions regarding the online attendance record for each student and grading of each student's tutorial performance at the end of the course.

Problem-based Learning Sessions

The Mechanics

1. Make introductions.
2. Hand out the first page of the case.
3. Participants read aloud the case one page at a time.
4. The group identifies the facts, clarifies definitions and terms, and generates hypotheses and learning agenda.
5. Discuss concepts using participant-generated diagrams on a blackboard.
6. Questions from discussion leader and participants guide the discussion.
7. Participants request the next page of the case after sufficient discussion.
8. The discussion leader summarizes the session with the closure schematic or colorful "placemat."

A Blueprint

If the goal of the session is to learn as much as possible, then it is preferable to hand out the objectives and initial pages of the case before the session, to maximize preparation and participation. If the goal of the session is to see a group's ability to dissect a mystery case and come up with the answers using teamwork and group knowledge, without prior preparation, then the pages may be handed out as the case unfolds in the actual session. Traditionally, one student volunteers to read the case aloud, one page at a time, so that each student has the facts fresh in mind as the cooperative learning begins. The discussion leader has all visual aids ready at hand. Although it is beneficial to the smooth running of the tutorial to have a predetermined series of questions to bring out important concepts during the discussion, the leader may not use many or all of these questions, but rather use others that come to mind to help amplify and guide the discussion. Questions may be used to move the discussion from one topic to another to complete the discussion of important points. Faculty should prepare a five-minute summary, based on the stated objectives for the session, and study the given closure schematic to illustrate the concepts, or create one of their own or have the students create this for the group's understanding of essential concepts. The discussion leader may wish to summarize the discussion at certain points during the session, but enough time should be left for a final summary using a closure schematic, which may consist of definitions, diagrams, algorithms, or an amalgam of line drawings, pathology photomicrographs, endoscopic photographs, and illustrative figures or tables from classic journal articles, which serve to illuminate the discussion's key points and touch on important but to some students difficult to grasp concepts (see fig. 7.3). Students in the gastrointestinal pathophysiology course began to call the 11 x 17 inch colorful closure schematics *placemats* because of their resemblance to an actual tablemats, and the term stuck. The original idea for a closure schematic in teaching scientific material comes from Prof. Bruce Greenwald (1991).

The weekly one-hour faculty development tutor meetings during the course emphasize the upcoming case content as well as tutorial dynamics, visual aid review, and mechanics. At these sessions, each tutor is asked to share any difficulties or triumphs of his or her group with the other tutors. There are generally twenty-two to twenty-four tutors for the overall class of some one hundred seventy students on the New Pathway curriculum.

The meetings are fast paced and well attended. They begin with each tutor's description of his or her tutorial dynamics and the group's discussion of cross-cultural care triggers. The focus then shifts to the goal of making each tutor a content expert on the current tutorial material and the coming week's tutorial material. To accomplish this, I lead an intensive review of the major concepts, schematics, and tutorial slides. The meeting starts and ends on time (7–7:50 a.m.), with a minimum of announcements and distractions from the main goals: my listening to each tutor, to help him or her manage the tutorial group successfully, and my teaching them essential content expertise.

Give Out Objectives Beforehand

Over the years, it has become clear that the better-prepared students get more out of tutorial. Therefore, we now reiterate the objectives for each day's tutorial session at least one day ahead as well as give out or post online the pertinent case pages. The students prepare by reading relevant background textbooks and the required journal articles. The clearly written objectives cover all the pertinent pathophysiologic points to be discussed and guide the tutor's questions so that the tutorial covers the necessary material.

For the small-group sessions and the pathology laboratories, the leader gives out either objectives or questions beforehand. For their part in making the session productive, students are expected to have reviewed the objectives, required journal articles, and background pathophysiology ahead of time.

Here are three objectives for a tutorial that covers diarrhea, malabsorption, and maldigestion, taken from a tutorial case of Crohn disease that initially presents as infectious diarrhea:

1.   Explain the handling of salt and water by the small and large intestines.
2.   Describe fat absorption by the small intestine.
3.   Define the term choleretic diarrhea and recognize why it occurs.

Course Organization and Logical Progression with Built-in Reiteration and Review

The underlying formula for successful preclinical teaching was described in the earlier section of this chapter under *F,* for *formula.* I will elaborate on this formula now.

Exposition is followed by *exploration, reiteration,* and *review.* In practical terms, this means that the knowledge the students need is presented in a lecture format or small-group session. Then the students explore that knowledge in the setting of a real-life paper or Web case that has built-in opportunities to discuss the necessary concepts. The exploration may take the form of a group discussion, with explanatory diagrams put up on the blackboard, along with readings from textbooks, journal articles, queries to experts, and further discussion with the group after more background research has been done. The reiteration is accomplished by having different faculty members, with different interests and different strengths, bring out the same topic in multiple sessions. Review sessions are given once weekly to make sure that the major concepts are solidified in the students' understanding before moving on to the next organ group.

The seven organs in the gastrointestinal and hepatobiliary system are taught in the following sequence:

Week 1: Esophagus, stomach (two days)
Week 2: Small and large intestine, pancreas (four days)
Week 3: Liver, biliary system (four days)

Multiple teaching venues help to clarify each of the major pathophysiologic concepts. For instance, if the objective is to delineate the multiple mechanisms causing diarrhea, these mechanisms are taught in:

1. Separate lectures on diarrhea, infections of the gastrointestinal tract, and inflammatory bowel disease
2. A three-day tutorial problem-based learning case discussing infectious diarrhea, lactase deficiency diarrhea, diarrhea due to inflammatory bowel disease, bile salt diarrhea, fatty acid diarrhea, bacterial overgrowth diarrhea, osmotic and exudative diarrhea, and diarrhea due to celiac disease
3. Journal articles that focus on celiac disease, *Clostridium difficile* infection, and inflammatory bowel disease
4. A pathology lecture that reviews the differences between ulcerative colitis and Crohn disease and that covers ischemic colitis
5. A pathology laboratory that reviews Crohn disease and ulcerative colitis
6. Web-based cases that include a virtual case of celiac disease and multimedia cases of ischemic colitis and *E. coli* 0157:H7
7. Weekly Friday reviews of pathophysiologic concepts, in which the mechanisms of water and salt absorption by the small and large intestine and concepts of maldigestion versus malabsorption are delineated and explained.
8. A final course review, in which the mechanisms for infectious and noninfectious diarrhea are enumerated and explained, so they are clear before the final exam.

The medical school computer system (My Courses) permits excellent communication and posting of resources (Cook et al. 2008). Thus, all tutorial objectives are conveyed to the students via the Web site. In addition, all faculty guides and slides for the small sessions, including the pathology laboratories, are placed on the Web to appear after the session has ended. All lectures and review sessions are videotaped and are accessible for viewing twenty-four hours a day. Numerous Web-based cases, most of which have an interactive component, such as the Virtual Patient cases or multimedia cases, are available to supplement the curriculum in areas that are covered only briefly in lectures, such as appendicitis, colonic volvulus, and Hirschprung disease. Other Web-based cases reinforce concepts that are already emphasized in the course, such as infectious diarrhea due to *E. coli* O157:H7, ischemic bowel disease, acute cholecystitis, diverticulitis, NSAID gastritis, *Helicobacter pylori* gastritis, and Crohn disease (fig. 7.4).

✄ TEACHING TIPS

1. Faculty members need to be trained in both content and methods to effectively teach in a problem-based curriculum.
2. The rationale behind even the simplest exercise should be transparent; students need to know what the goals are to be confident that they can achieve them by completing the tasks that you, as the course director or curriculum creator, have devised.
3. The objectives for each session need to be clear, be concise, and reflect the course goals.
4. The course should be well organized and have a logical progression.
5. The sequence of exposition, exploration, reiteration, and review provides a consistent and logical framework for students to master large amounts of material in a short time.
6. A Web-based source of additional materials and study aids along with answer keys and interactive questions is invaluable.
7. The Web site encourages strong organization by permitting regular reminders of objectives and required readings. It ties the faculty and students together in a quest for better communication of teaching goals because both faculty and students know the objectives ahead of time.
8. A dedicated course manager or administrator who schedules sessions and room assignments, is responsible for publishing the syllabus in a timely fashion, and provides answers to organizational problems is essential for a smooth-running course.

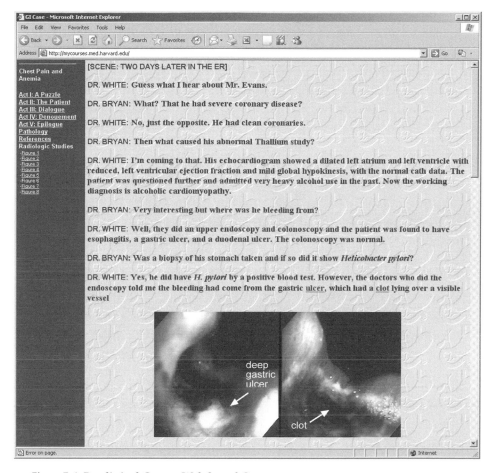

Figure 7.4. **Preclinical Course Web-based Case**
Encourage students to read online case material that reiterates concepts in the course or breaks new ground. Case depicted is "Chest Pain and Anemia in a Middle-Aged Man: A Mystery in Five Acts," by Kitt Shaffer, Helen Shields, and Melissa Upton. The creation of this case was funded by an education grant from Harvard Medical School in 1998–99.

Source: Harvard Medical School Intranet Web site. Copyright 1999 President and Fellows of Harvard College. Reprinted with permission of Harvard Medical School.

9. The creation of a teaching fellow position permits fellows-in-training to improve their teaching skills before accepting a faculty position and is a source of inspiration, new ideas, and enthusiasm for the course director.

Tutoring in a Preclinical Course

I had been a course director for eight years and a tutor for more than ten years when I was put on the Committee for Experienced Tutors by Dr. Daniel Federman, dean of Medical Education. The major function of this committee was to provide twice-yearly faculty development sessions for tutors who wished to learn more about small-group teaching methods. Another member of the committee, David Golan, MD, PhD, suggested that a professor from Harvard Business School be our keynote speaker because he was interested in the similarities and differences between the case-based methods used at the business school, the medical school, and the law school. As I sat and listened to Prof. David Garvin's electrifying presentation on the case method at the business school, I knew that I wanted to try to bring some of these methods to the medical school. We began to use three teaching strategies from the business school in our tutorial: the use of questions throughout the tutorial by the tutor, an end-of-tutorial summary given by the tutor, and a closure schematic, or "placemat" (see fig. 7.3). Several years ago, Dr. Alexander Carbo's tutorial group began calling the closure schematics *placemats* because they resemble colorful and attractive 11 x 17 inch placemats. The nickname has stuck.

On the first day, begin by introducing yourself. Tell the students where you are from geographically and mention a hobby. Then ask them where they come from and ask then to name an interest or a hobby. This gets away from which college they attended, their honors, scholarships or global policy initiatives, and puts the students and tutor on a more even footing as the tutorial begins.

Begin on time, even if only one student in your group is there. This means arriving fifteen to thirty minutes early to get books, case pages, and schematics ready before the tutorial starts, regardless of bad weather. If students come late, your having started on time will make them aware that the learning starts on time. Take the latecomers aside at the end of this tutorial. Ask the reason for the lateness. Was it bus, alarm clock, late night studying, childcare? Let the student know that you expect him or her to fix whatever the problem is, as a matter of professionalism, and remind the student to be on time for the next session.

End your session on time. The students, no matter how enthusiastic, resent any intrusion into their free time for coffee or messaging before their next class/lab/lecture. Be careful to note that the ending time of the tutorial may differ for different dates. Carefully follow the course calendar's time frames. Ask one of the students to remind you when you are five to ten minutes from the end.

Prepare well for each session. Make a list of potential questions at the bottom of each case page. Rehearse the end-of-tutorial summary. If you are using a schematic, review the concepts carefully. Read the references that will explain each concept. Remember to hand out the diagram/schematic as you begin your summary so that students can follow along.

Let the group do the work, but do ask guiding questions to direct the discussion, to assure that it covers the pathophysiologic mechanisms they are responsible for.

Listen intently to the tutorial discussion and observe the body language of the participants and the group dynamics. I generally do not jot down notes when I am tutoring until after the session has ended and the students have gone. My note taking may detract from the group's discussion. When I am alone, I will do a shorthand notation in a grid that I make up before the start of the first session (see fig. 6.2). The grid has each student's name and a box for brief comments, such as "went to blackboard for acid secretion diagram," etc., and the date of tutorial. I use this as a reminder of what the student did. The comments and shorthand will provide you with sufficient examples or trends to readily fill in the evaluation form on each student at the end of the course. In addition, when you meet with each student for feedback, it will be easier to speak to him or her with chapter and verse of contributions to tutorial and dates.

Encourage students to go to the blackboard to clarify and diagram important concepts, but do not go there yourself; in tutorial, the blackboard is usually considered the students' domain.

Bring in additional materials—x-rays, references, photos—to expand or clarify a point.

Be pleasant, relaxed, but alert and enthusiastic. The group will reflect your mood.

Be careful about bringing into the tutorial any troubles or deadlines that you may have weighing on your mind. The students will pick this up and feel for you rather than learning what you are trying to teach. Your business is best left outside the classroom except in controlled ways, when you give out specific information about your background, hobbies, family, or education.

Ask for feedback on the tutorial at the end of each of the first few sessions. You can alter your style if you hear that the students wish you would speak more, be quieter, or ask more questions. You may also hear that some are annoyed by the dominance of a few students or annoyed by the lack of participation of others. These matters need to be addressed immediately within the group. Be careful not to address the group's problems with just one or two students; this looks to the other students like teacher favoritism.

Hand out the materials for the next day's discussion at the end of the tutorial. I frequently ask one of the first students to arrive that day to remind me to hand out the next part of the case. I also put all handouts down in front of me, so it is almost impossible for me to forget to hand them out at the end of the tutorial.

Make time to view exhibits that are essential to the case. Ask another student to remind you when you said you wanted to view the visuals. Ask the students when they would prefer to view slide materials on the plasma screen and take a vote if the group is clearly divided on when to view the ancillary images for the case.

Try to engage the quiet student and modulate the dominant student. Speak with both types of student as soon as possible at the end of the tutorial. Solicit their honest views on how the tutorial is working as a learning experience for them. This one-on-one discussion is your best opportunity to modulate the dominant student and to encourage the quiet students to speak up. I often recognize dominant students as great contributors but let them know that I believe their exceptionally strong knowledge base is shutting off discussion for other students. I ask these students to hold information back and let others have the floor, because I already know that they know the answer. With quiet students, I ask which material they wish to be the expert on. We prearrange a short topic discussion of the student's choice. I will look at them when the topic logically comes up in the tutorial, giving them the subtle signal to speak about the prepared material. This method usually works to get the student involved as a contributing, if not spontaneous, member of the group.

Obtain each student's cell phone number or home phone number (with answering machine) at the beginning of the first session and give the tutorial group all of your phone numbers and your business card. This exchange of phone numbers will prove useful if you or a student is late, due to bad weather conditions, car problems, or illness. Their calling you saves you from unexplained absences in tutorial and feedback sessions.

Schedule midcourse feedback meetings as early as possible after the first few tutorials to let each student know how he or she is doing. Tell students at the beginning of your session how much you appreciate their participation and give an example or examples from your grid of what they have done to impress you. Memorize the examples you have from your grid; do not show the student the grid. Remembering the examples establishes you as caring about the student's contributions. You will start off on the right foot. After this, you may wish to ask the students to comment on the tutorial and if it is working for them. Give negative feedback about tardiness or lack of preparation, if this is occurring. Otherwise, students will be unhappy when these items appear in the tutorial evaluation without your having called it specifically to their attention.

Use any type of food, fruit, crackers, snack, or drink as an icebreaker at tutorials. Conversation flows better when both students and faculty are not hungry.

At the last tutorial, consider bringing in breakfast, lunch, or dinner. Depending on how close you and the group have grown, you may wish to ask the group to go out for a meal or come to your home. Ask at least a week ahead of time what the students would like to do so that each of you can plan for the meal or get-together. If you have had a good time tutoring, it is wise to do something to recognize the significance of your learning together. Note how pleased you are to have been a member of the teaching faculty. This creates a good atmosphere for making the final push to learn the content of the course before the final exam.

Using your grid, complete your evaluations of each student within two weeks after the course ends.

Table 7.2 lists questions to ask yourself before you begin tutoring.

✂ TEACHING TIPS

1. Begin on time. This means arriving fifteen to thirty minutes early to get books, case pages, and schematics out of the locker before the tutorial begins.
2. End on time.

Table 7.2.   Questions to Ask before You Begin Tutoring

1. Am I ready to spend the time necessary to learn the material well enough to teach it with clarity? If the answer is no, then consider backing out immediately rather than having a fiasco on your teaching record.
2. What am I hoping to gain from the experience: a credit for my CV, a relationship with students that is more fun than that on the wards, instruction in small-group teaching techniques, or enjoyment of the camaraderie of teaching with a group of teachers?
3. Am I open to learning new approaches to small-group teaching?
4. Can I attend each of the faculty development sessions so that I maximize my chances of being successful with my group?
5. Have I blocked my time with my secretary, the department chair, and the department administrators so that they know my income production may be significantly lower during this time?
6. Am I enthusiastic enough about my teaching assignment to put up with the loss of income and with patients who resent my not being as available during teaching assignment times?
7. Have I alerted patients that I will not be as available during those weeks?
8. Am I tutoring in the hopes of getting a recommendation letter from the course director for my upcoming promotion to assistant or associate professor?
9. Am I tutoring in the hopes of being noticed by the senior faculty as a possible teacher for other assignments in the future?
10. Are there specific tutoring awards that I should strive for?

3. Prepare well for each session:

   a. Make a list of potential questions at the bottom of each case page.
   b. Rehearse the end-of-tutorial summary.
   c. If you are using a closure schematic, review it carefully. Do not forget to hand out the schematics to each student before beginning the summary.

4. Let the group do the work. Use guiding questions to make sure that the discussion covers the pathophysiologic mechanisms on the daily schematic.
5. Listen intently to the tutorial discussion and observe the body language of the participants and the group dynamics. Make a note to yourself regarding each student's participation/contribution at the end of each tutorial session. This will make your evaluations and feedback sessions with them easier.
6. Encourage students to go to the blackboard to clarify and diagram important concepts. Never go to the blackboard; this is the student's domain in tutorial.

7. Bring additional materials, such as x-rays, endoscopic photos, or articles, if you wish to clarify or expand a point.

8. Be pleasant and relaxed but alert and enthusiastic. The group will reflect your mood.

9. Ask for feedback on your and the group's performance at the end of each day of the first week's tutorials

10. Do not forget to hand out the case pages for the next day's discussion at the end of each tutorial.

11. View tutorial slides with your group on the plasma screen.

12. Try to engage the quiet student and modulate the dominant student. Speak with either type of student as soon as possible at the end of a tutorial session so that he or she may change the behavior.

13. Schedule midcourse feedback meetings during the second week for ten-minute intervals before tutorial begins. Let each student know how much you appreciate his or her participation and give an example of what each student has done.

14. Obtain each student's cell phone number at the beginning of the first session and give each of them your phone number. This will be useful for bad weather conditions, car problems, illness, and unexplained absences or missed feedback sessions.

15. Use any type of food or drink as a good icebreaker.

16. Consider bringing in a farewell breakfast or taking your group to lunch or dinner after the course is over.

17. Volunteer to help at the end of the course to grade exams; you will gain the appreciation of the course director and meet other teachers you may not know.

18. Complete your tutorial students' evaluations within two weeks after the end of tutorial. This requirement will not go away, and it gets harder and harder to complete the evaluations as time goes on because your memory of events and students' performance in the tutorial will fade. Do it early and make it easier for yourself.

Mini-cases and Focused Discussions

I have modified only slightly the directions for mini-cases and focused discussions that were created by Dr. Miriam S. Wetzel in the mid-1990s and explained to me by Dr. Wetzel when I took over as course director for the gastrointestinal pathophysiology course. Mini-cases and focused discussions are small-group sessions for twelve to forty people that usually last an hour but may run for as long as an hour and three quarters. Mini-cases are distinguished from focused discussions. The mini-case has questions that, ideally, the students look over before the session and postulate answers to, based on their reading of the lecture material and required references for the week or by going to the lecture before the session. Focused discussions, in contrast, have objectives rather than questions (fig. 7.5). Topics are more complex and usually have not been covered in lecture or tutorial and therefore do not lend themselves as well to an interactive session. Instead, the faculty member gives a succinct lecture that covers the objectives, striving for a less interactive session because the students do not have much prior knowledge of the complex material.

In either type of small-group discussion, you are considered an expert who will enlighten the group and provide clear explanations of answers to questions and summaries of the objectives. In our gastrointestinal pathophysiology course, for instance, we relegate the complex subjects—the enteric nervous system and the pathogenesis of irritable bowel, the genetics of colon cancer and familial colon cancer syndromes and polyps, and the genetic pathogenesis of hemochromatosis—to the more labor-intensive focused discussions by faculty, whereas the more readily grasped subjects—lower esophageal

- Explain the role of fundus, antrum, pylorus, gastric pacemaker, and migrating motor complex in gastric emptying.
- Differentiate between the normal gastric emptying of liquids and solids.
- Distinguish mechanical obstruction versus non-mechanical causes of delayed gastric emptying.
- Describe the defects found in diabetic gastroparesis patients that contribute to their gastric emptying problems.

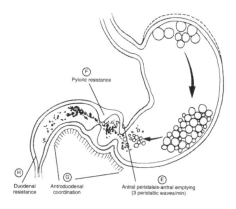

Figure 7.5. **Example of Objectives: One-Hour Small-Group Session on Gastric Emptying**
Indicate what you expect to accomplish in the one-hour session. Use an action verb to begin each objective. Objectives for a focused discussion on gastric emptying are listed, with a diagram showing the later phases of gastric emptying.
Illustration source: Koch 1993, 163. Reprinted, with permission, from *Atlas of Gastrointestinal Motility in Health and* Disease, ed. Marvin M. Schuster (Baltimore: Williams & Wilkins, 1993).

Table 7.3. Questions to Ask before You Begin Preparing for Mini-cases and Focused Discussions

1. What are the consequences of doing well?
2. What are the consequences of doing poorly?
3. Do I want to be asked to come back?
4. Do I want never to be asked back?
5. Could doing well lead to other opportunities?
6. Am I going to attend all of the faculty-development sessions offered for the group I am teaching?
7. What are the evaluations based on? May I see an evaluation sheet before I begin?
8. Who are my co-teachers? Are they likely to help me if they have done it before?

sphincter pressure, high (achalasia) or low (scleroderma), acute pancreatitis, mesenteric ischemia, extrahepatic versus intrahepatic jaundice, bilirubin metabolism, and gallstone formation—are discussed in an interactive manner in mini-case sessions, where a specific lecture on the topic precedes a small-group session. Faculty who are successful prepare intensively before the session with the references, lecture materials, and slides, which we provide approximately a month in advance. They are careful about the time allotment and ask questions of themselves and others until they are sure they have mastered the material and can clearly and succinctly explain it.

Because the students expect you to be an expert in the area, prepare extensively and rehearse your presentation beforehand. Review the slides you have been given, and ask if you may add some of your own. Usually the course director is delighted to have you introduce new and often better visual images as long as you cover the main points of the pathophysiology. I will frequently ask the faculty member to substitute his or her slides for our old set and give this faculty member credit by putting his or her name on the next year's official slide set. Being enthusiastic and responsive to the students during the session is essential to getting a good grade.

Table 7.3 lists questions to ask yourself before you begin preparing for mini-cases and focused discussions.

Mechanics of a sixty-minute mini-case session with two problem-based cases:

- Case read by students, followed by the faculty member's interactive discussion with students of each case's questions (approximate time: ten to fifteen minutes).
- Faculty member gives exposition of necessary background anatomy

and physiology, as well as pertinent pathophysiologic points, using blackboard or slides (approximate time: ten to fifteen minutes).

- Faculty member summarizes major take-home message at the end of each case or at the end of both cases (approximate time: one to five minutes).
- The guide and slides for each case are made available on the medical school Web site immediately after the session finishes for the students to review the important points of each presentation. This acts as a safety net for faculty who do not cover all the material.

Mechanics of a sixty-minute session with one topic:

1. Thirty to forty minutes: Reading of case by students followed by an interactive discussion of the case and objectives by students and faculty member. The blackboard, slides, x-rays, or other teaching aids may be used for the exposition of necessary basic anatomy and physiology, as well as pertinent pathophysiologic points by the faculty member.
2. Ten to twenty minutes: Reiteration and review of important points by faculty member. Make sure you cover the answers to each objective (see fig. 7.5). I assign one student to be my objective keeper and another to be the timer, who holds up a hand when thirty minutes have passed.
3. The guide and slides for each case are made available on the medical school Web site immediately after the session ends for the students to review the important points of each presentation. This acts as a safety net for faculty members who do not cover all the material.

✂ TEACHING TIPS

1. Be kind and connect with your audience of fifteen to twenty students. Start on time, even if only one or two students are present.

   a. Read out loud ahead of time the students' names, which you should receive along with your room assignment. Ask for your students' names ahead of time to practice pronouncing them.
   b. Introduce yourself and ask each student's name and note his or her seating position.
   c. Write your name and institution (phone, e-mail address) on the blackboard.

2. Arrange the seats in a semicircle around you if you are in a large room. Do not allow students to sit in areas where they cannot be seen, as this may detract from the teaching presentation and distract other students, if these students begin to whisper.

3. Arrive fifteen to thirty minutes early to set up your slides in the projector, preview them, clean the blackboard, and draw diagrams or list important points on the blackboard.

4. Use the students' names when calling on them to answer questions or discuss objectives.

5. Stand up for your presentation and move around a bit, with energy and enthusiasm. Make your session fun and interactive.

6. Ask one of the students to tell you when half the allotted time is up. Ask another student to ensure that all objectives are covered (focused discussions).

7. You are evaluated on the clarity of your presentation and on your ability to connect with the students. The students enjoy an enthusiastic and lively presentation, so plan your session accordingly. Consistently move the session along while explaining, reiterating, and reviewing concepts and important terms at every possible juncture. Use the blackboard to expand the understanding of concepts. I prefer to use the blackboard early in my presentations and to use the slides as a summary. The exception to this suggestion is when an x-ray is essential to the case diagnosis and needs to be shown during the case reading.

8. Review your teaching materials carefully and strengthen any areas of weakness for the pathophysiologic concepts you are to teach.

9. Make the material your own and put your own spin on it. Have a detailed lesson plan worked out in mind and on paper. Use index cards as memory prompts during the presentation. A step-by-step approach to understanding the pathophysiology of the illnesses described will impress your audience. If no faculty-development sessions are offered, then find out who did well the prior year or teaching cycle and ask him or her how to do well. Be wary of taking the advice of the cynical teacher who is repeating the teaching exercise only because it is fulfilling a required teaching obligation. This person could steer you wrong and have you preparing little, preferring to "wing it." Teaching this session well is clearly not important for this person's career track, but it may be important for yours.

10. Do not be sidetracked by student questions that are not germane to un-

derstanding the essential pathophysiologic concepts. Instead, volunteer to answer those questions from a particular student at the end. The other students will appreciate your staying on track.

11. Wind down each case with a clear summary of pathophysiology using slides or the blackboard. Do not be afraid to repeat yourself. Repetition of important points is appreciated. If you are running short on time, do not worry about skipping some of the material or even slides. The tutor guide and slides may be available to students following each session. If they are not, ask the course director if you can send your group your slide set and a summary because you did not finish the material. However, I find that when I skip material because time is running out, my evaluations suffer.

12. Practice in advance the timing of your session, which will include having the students read the case, answer the questions for mini-cases, understand the objectives for focused discussions, and view the slides.

13. End on time; otherwise, the students will begin to leave before you are finished.

14. Remember that the students will evaluate your teaching. Several of our mini-case and focused discussion leaders have been nominated for or have received teaching awards.

15. Know that understanding pathophysiologic concepts, not clinical medicine, should be the major goal of all preclinical pathophysiology teaching sessions.

16. Give feedback and make suggestions to your course director regarding the session.

Lecturing in a Preclinical Course

Fewer lectures are given nowadays in medical schools because many schools have turned to small-group problem-based learning methods. Therefore, to be asked to lecture in a preclinical medical school course is considered a prize or plum assignment. Unfortunately, I too often hear negative comments from students about the lectures given in the preclinical courses. The major problem appears to be a "disconnect" between the material the students feel should be covered and what is covered. Lecturers require individual instructions on content, suggested delivery, and lecture note format. The lecturer needs to know the course syllabus, how his or her content piece fits into the fabric of the course, the objectives of the course for the material he or she is invited to cover. The course fabric should be tightly woven so that each lecture is an important and integral part of the seamless teaching. Specific details of what should be taught are essential to impart to the lecturer if this assignment is to be successfully fulfilled. Course objectives and an old syllabus should be shared with the lecturer, giving him or her an idea of the note format as well as the desired level to pitch the content.

✂ TEACHING TIPS

1. Your lecture is part of a tightly woven course fabric; do not lecture without knowing the rest of the course fabric and where your lecture fits in.

2. Obtain course objectives, problem-based learning cases, mini-cases and focused discussion cases, old lecture notes from the prior lecturer, as well as pathology laboratory cases before you write your lecture notes and make your slides; you will never regret knowing what is covered in other venues of the same course.

3. Medical students often give high marks to lecturers whose notes are written out in paragraph form, particularly if an excellent textbook is not available on the subject. Students then rely on the lecture notes as a complete source of knowledge.

4. Spend time creating your lecture notes and reference lists; the effort will not be wasted.

5. Be sure to ask what required references and book chapters are being used for the course, in case one or more of them pertains to your talk. Know this material well and weave it into your talk.

6. Contact the audiovisual department if you expect to run a video, DVD, or other more sophisticated presentation during your lecture to avoid having a disaster at the podium; at a minimum, send your presentation ahead to the administrator of the course and make sure he or she can open it and view it with no difficulty.

7. Bring your lecture on a memory stick as a backup in case something is wrong with the copy you sent; the biggest problems with delivery are having too many slides for the time allotted, followed by audiovisual glitches.

8. Make sure you arrive thirty minutes before your lecture to view the auditorium, check your presentation, and familiarize yourself with the podium controls, pointer, and slide advancer.

9. If a lecture is going on before yours, use this time to observe the audience of medical students, noting their body language and questions for

the lecturer. As soon as the lecture preceding yours is finished, walk to the podium so that the microphone can be placed on your jacket; wearing a jacket with pockets helps with stowing away the portable microphone battery pack.

10. Consider coming the week before your lecture to listen and observe another lecture in the same course, or even a different course, to gain an idea of the venue, the class attitude, and what seems to work best.

11. Smile at the student audience as the course director introduces you; you will gain good will at the outset.

12. Speak clearly and slowly because part of the class will view your lecture online as a video.

13. If few students come to your lecture, do not be rattled; they have their priorities. A great lecture this year may change your audience size next year because of the underground student rating system that frequently prevails in medical schools.

14. If you are a yearly lecturer and few students come to your lecture, you may wish to ask for the verbatim comments of the students from the year before, if the course director has not already given them to you. Occasionally, a mediocre lecturer is kept in the lineup just because no one else is capable of lecturing on the specific topic. You do not have to be that mediocre lecturer.

15. Students like clarity, logic, relevance, excellent and colorful visuals, a good summary, and "take-away points" in the lecture itself.

16. Watch for the too-many-slides phenomenon, a trap that is easy to fall into; one slide per minute or minute and a half is a good rule.
    Few slides are so essential that you need to ruin your lecture evaluations by stuffing them into too short a time.

17. Reiterate and review within your lecture format your important points; less is more. Your lecture notes can be the more, while your lecture should be the less.

18. Rotate your head; get out from behind the podium; ask for the portable microphone ahead of time. Students enjoy a lecturer who moves about and fixes his or her gaze on the entire audience in a sweeping motion.

19. Leave time for questions; plan to stay afterward to answer more questions, because some students may be too shy to ask when you are speaking. You may need to step outside the auditorium to continue answering questions from students if another lecture is about to begin.

20. Ask the course director how your lecture went; if the course director was not there, ask for your written evaluations when the director receives them.

21. Students ask that industry conflicts of interest be displayed; your first slide should indicate whether you have conflicts of interest and what organizations or companies they are with.

22. Arrogance, sarcasm, and gender jokes are never appreciated; don't go there.

23. Respect the students; pretend you are being paid a great deal of money for this lecture, for which you may receive no compensation. Remember how wonderful great lecturers seemed when you were a medical student. They took on the status of movie stars if they could illuminate dark areas of neurology, nephrology, cardiology, or other hard-won concepts.

24. If your evaluations are poor, ask the course director for one more try, with input from him or her to help guide you toward success. Delivery is important; if this is the problem, get a coach to help you with public speaking, diction, poise, and phrasing—all essential parts of any academic physician's career skill set.

✂ TAKE-HOME POINTS

- Prepare and deliver your lecture as if you are being paid; it is an honor to teach medical students.
- Know where your content fits into to the whole course plan; if this information is not volunteered, go after it.
- Clarity, logic, and relevance are prized much more than completeness; this is not postgraduate lecturing, in which the material is relatively familiar. Here the material is foreign and can be unsettling to the student audience unless presented in easy-to-grasp sections.
- Hand in both lecture notes and slides to be distributed or downloaded before the lecture so that students can write next to the slides extra information from the lecture.
- Build reiteration and review into your lecture; you can never do enough of this if the subject is new and complex for the students.
- Leave time for questions; some students will wish to ask you individually after the lecture.

CHAPTER EIGHT

Clinical Teaching

- *What preparations are necessary to be an excellent teaching-attending physician on the ward in-patient service?*
- *How do I give my best to the patients and their need for correct decisions and to the residents and their learning needs?*
- *How can I use evidence-based medicine in my teaching sessions?*
- *How do I make bedside rounds fun and educational?*
- *What methods maximize my group's functioning as a team?*
- *What are potential pitfalls for a specialty consult attending physician?*
- *How do I effectively manage my time with patients and my teaching as an ambulatory attending physician?*

Inpatient Teaching

Methods and Attitudes for Success as an Attending Physician

House staff, students, and fellows want to gain the experience and knowledge that attending physicians have. In addition, they desire direct feedback about their clinical skills. As the attending, you need to impart experience, knowledge, and feedback in an engaging and appealing manner, on rounds and at the bedside. You also need to focus on quality in medical care, systems-based practice, and patient safety (Fitzgibbons et al. 2006). You want to be both great and memorable in a short space of time. Put yourself in your team members' shoes. They are generally too busy or too tired to enjoy attending rounds, even though they are ostensibly in residency to learn. Creating good will early in your rotation will help your ultimate job of molding their knowledge, attitudes, skills, and behaviors. Make rounds interesting, fun, informative, and evidence based. Avoid being a drag on the team's efficiency. One way to accomplish this is to work closely with the junior or senior resident who is head of your house-staff team. Use this person to guide your efforts, at least initially. If he or she is leading you correctly, you will know by the smiles and nods of approval as you touch on subjects that the head resident has suggested that the group wishes to hear about. If rounds are faltering, feel and see this, and make adjustments. Make sure you find out what the group wants from you and try to adjust immediately.

The residents and students are your charges to teach, evaluate, and supervise, as well as your team to consult (Steinmann et al. 2009). Respect them as your peripheral brain. Do not try to be head honcho running the show with no input from them. They will be bored, rather than engaged. Use their computer skills and fund of knowledge as talents to be brought to the consulting table, along with your clinical wisdom, years of experience, and acknowledged expertise.

The patients are also your legal responsibility, if you are not just the teaching-attending but also the attending of record. The greatest challenge that the teaching-attending faces is balancing two very different needs: the need to assure that patients receive high-quality care, making your decisions transparent so that others can learn from you, and the need to teach and supervise residents and medical students so that their clinical skills and thinking ability are developed and evaluated while not compromising patient care (Irby 1992). As J. Willis Hurst (1999) notes, "true teachers recognize the importance of basic science to clinical medicine" (33), and "true teachers study" (38).

Details of practical preparation mark the difference between a successful teaching-attending experience and a frustrating one. Being a great attending means freeing up your schedule for teaching. This means having your secretary or administrator block out your schedule appropriately and conservatively as soon as you are notified that you are the attending for a block of time. Blocking your schedule will get you to rounds on time, give you time for preparation, and leave you not dreading attending because of the havoc it plays with your clinical schedule. Conflict between duties as an attending and your administrative and patient responsibilities is a major reason for poor performance as an attending and for not wanting to be a teaching-attending again. Agree to cancel your clinics and procedures or surgery slots during your one- or two-week teaching-attending time and lose the income; it is impossible to serve two masters at once. Your clinical patients must take a back seat to your teaching obligations unless they have emergencies during the time you are teaching.

It is wise to announce the dates of your teaching-attending duties to each patient who calls to schedule during the months before your teaching obligation. This lets patients know early on that you will devote your time primarily to another essential activity, that of teaching. My administrator and I take the opportunity to tell each patient that I am seeing or speaking with that I am the attending each September on the inpatient gastrointestinal consult service at my hospital. The patients are alerted well in advance and reassured that, if an emergency arises, I will either see them before or after I finish teaching or have them seen by another physician. I try not to schedule any nonemergent endoscopic procedures or clinic visits, leaving me free to focus on the inpatient service and my teaching and patient care responsibilities. Emergencies do occur among my own outpatients, but the number of patients who need to be seen during my attending time is dramatically reduced. I ask my administrator to field calls while I am in attending rounds. If an emergency arises, then I or another attending covering me takes the call. If I cannot see the patient in clinic because of rounds, he or she will be seen by another attending or by an emergency room physician. I will check up with the patient in person or by phone later that evening or the next day.

When I teach on the general medicine service, I turn off my beeper during rounds so that I will not be interrupted. Another faculty member from my practice takes emergency calls while my secretary fields the nonemergency calls. Having to take emergency calls is a distraction for those trying to learn from you and causes your mind to switch to a different direction from teaching. Your team does not learn anything useful from your having to turn your back on them to answer calls. When I make specialty rounds with the gastrointestinal fellow, I leave my beeper on, however, because the pages I receive may relate to the patients we are seeing. I ask my administrator to avoid paging me during rounds. I will return all calls after rounds and late into the evenings when I am attending.

Try to avoid having deadlines for projects, grants, and major talks during clinical attending times. Complete your deadlines before you start attending. An excellent attending is able to look relaxed, interested, and ready to teach because his or her clinical and administrative responsibilities are minimized for that time period due to advance planning. Attending is like a marathon race; to run it successfully, you need to devote much time and energy to preparing for it.

Prepare at an intellectual level. Reichsman, Browning, and Hinshaw (1964, 161) note that "the task faced by the clinical teacher is unique in the entire realm of clinical teaching. In no other field does the nature of the material demand of the teacher this degree of preparedness without preparation." How can you prepare to have your decisions under the microscope and open to challenge? You can read the major journals in your field. If you are attending on medicine, read the *New England Journal of Medicine* or *Annals of Internal Medicine*. On surgery, read the *American Journal of Surgery* or the *Annals of Surgery*. Are you aware of the innovations in your field and the latest advances in pharmacology and therapeutics? What are your opinions about controversial scientific and ethical problems in medicine? What short talks are you ready to give? Organize them in one place so that you can pull them out when you need them. Have a cache of teaching x-rays, slides, gross or pathologic findings, or endoscopic photos that you are ready to show on rounds at a moment's notice.

Use Evidence-based Medicine

Attending physicians should be enthusiastic and effective role models leading the way in the practice of evidence-based medicine, as defined and outlined by Dan Mayer in the book *Essential Evidence-Based Medicine* (2004), by the Evidence-Based Medicine Working Group (1992), and by Heneghan and Glasziou (2005) and Nicholson and Shieh (2005). Critical appraisal of the issues in patient-care management should be a central, pragmatic issue, not a tangential element of patient care. Bennett et al. (1987) showed years ago that critical appraisal skills of medical literature can be taught to medical students and that improvement can occur.

Use evidence-based medicine on rounds to help you identify proven therapies for patients. Evidence-based medicine has been defined as the conscientious, explicit, and judicious use of the best evidence in making decisions about the care of individual patients. The seven steps involved in evidence-based medicine are:

1. Design a clinical question to answer a clinical dilemma, including in the question the patient or patient population of interest, the intervention contemplated, the comparison between interventions, and the outcome of interest to your patient.
2. Research the medical literature for the best evidence that includes double-blind randomized placebo-controlled trials as well as meta-analyses for summarizing randomized controlled trials.
3. Learn to systematically evaluate the validity of the clinical evidence and the quantitative techniques for summarizing the evidence by

reading articles on how to access, evaluate, and interpret the medical literature.

4. Find the study that is best able to answer your question.
5. Do a critical appraisal of the study to determine its validity.
6. Examine how the results will help you in caring for your patient.
7. Evaluate the results of your intervention in your patient or patient population.

To summarize, good questions for the evidence-based medicine process involve patient, intervention, comparison, and outcome. Evidence-based medicine should be part of each physician's everyday life as well as part of a physician's commitment to lifelong learning. Inpatient teaching rounds is an excellent venue in which to encourage researching the medical literature to find the best evidence for a particular intervention and in which to critically appraise that evidence.

Equipment You Need for Rounds

Ready your clean white coats (tax deduction for laundry bills), long or short, depending on your hospital's style for an attending. Check your stethoscope's rubber tubing; it may need to be changed or you may need to get a new stethoscope. Consider investing in a better stethoscope before attending rounds start so that you can hear as many murmurs, rales, ronchi, wheezes, bruits, and friction rubs as possible on physical examinations during rounds. Be sure your nametag, with picture, is up to date and accessible on your coat. Patient and team members can readily see who you are and what department you represent. Wear comfortable shoes for the prolonged standing that occurs on rounds.

Keep a pocket-sized notebook in a side pocket to record the patient's name and medical record number sticker, along with the date you see the patient, major diagnoses, and the date of your initial note and progress notes. These facts help for billing chores, but they also provide a permanent record of patients with interesting histories or physical findings for future teaching. Put 3 x 5 inch or 5 x 7 inch index cards and pens in your upper pocket to write down a "to do" list for the next day's rounds, such as looking up a physical finding or an x-ray, or use an electronic planner or list maker. Whatever suits you best is fine; just do not forget to bring to rounds the next day what you promised the team. In your upper pocket, keep a short centimeter ruler, for measuring masses, liver size, and skin lesions, and a pocket flashlight, so you can see interesting physical findings in dimly lit patient rooms. Bring a covered coffee, tea, or other beverage of your choice to rounds to help you stay as sharp as possible. Eat breakfast if this helps you think clearly. Sufficient sleep, if possible, the night before is useful when you are presented with five complex cases in a row or even one befuddling case, with has extensive laboratory and x-ray data to evaluate, on rounds. Bring money to treat the team to coffee or tea occasionally. Bagels and cream cheese or donuts are much appreciated by the team, especially for Saturday or Sunday rounds. Consider treating the team at the end of your attending time to a coffee cake, pizza, or special dinner. Treating the team will not change either their opinion of you as a teacher or clinician or their grading of your attending abilities. Treat if you wish to thank your team for a job well done or want to know your team members better on a more personal level. Do not treat to improve your grades.

Set Expectations and Avoid Pitfalls

Ask ahead of time about the reputation of your team members. Forewarned is forearmed. Knowing the personalities and styles of the medical, surgical, or consult team you've been assigned to may help you do your job better or anticipate potential problems before they arise. Alternatively, you can decide to "wing it," hoping to bring out the best in the team members, no matter what their reputation. Medical students will rotate through, as well as visiting residents and medical students from other hospitals and medical schools; these people's personalities and styles will be unknown to you.

If you prefer not to have mystery cases presented to you, find out whom you should contact before the first attending rounds to learn what cases will be presented. Introducing yourself to the patient before rounds is also useful, if you want to have a picture in your mind of the patient as he or she is being presented. Remember that your team wants your best teaching. This means that if you do advance preparation, decide on your major teaching objectives for rounds, look up key articles to share, and ask insightful questions, your teaching will be memorable and to your credit.

On the first day, ask each person on the team what topics he or she would like you to cover during your time with them or give a list of topics that you excel at covering (canned talks). Write down what they say in your small, pocket-sized notebook, on your index cards, or in an electronic planner. Expect to cover at least 60 percent, if not more, of their wish list. Early on in your rotation, plot a strategy for how you will intercalate these minitalks into your rounds. Work with the junior or senior resident on your talk topics for the week. Ask the resident when it will be best to discuss the newest ways of colon cancer screening and the evidence for each, or the approach to the patient with atypical chest pain. Are there other pertinent topics? How long will your talk be? What day is best? One or more team members have generally gone to clinic, so do not hold up talks indefinitely to wait for the entire team to be there. But do pick the day that appears to have the least number of absentees. Otherwise, you lose opportunities to teach. Grab your teaching time whenever you can because if the service gets busy, there may be no time for you to teach. Each week I try to cover two topics that attendees have expressed interest in, but if the service is busy I sometimes get to cover only one. I may focus only on showing how to view an x-ray properly or go over a physical finding on a patient that I have noted was missed or misinterpreted or that needs a bit of discussion to appreciate its importance in shaping and prioritizing the differential diagnosis. Do not ask what talks you can give if this appears difficult or impossible for you to do. Rather, surprise your team one morning with a minitalk on a pertinent subject. This may be all you can do, but it will be appreciated.

As an alternative to minitalks, consider giving a discussion of how you got where you are and some lessons you have learned about career advancement. Let the team know that you are happy to meet with them individually or collectively to discuss career plans and offer advice for ten- or fifteen-minute periods before or after rounds. Most if not all residents, interns, and medical students in medicine and surgery appreciate getting advice from an interested attending on future goals and prospects. Some of these team members will ask you for recommendations for residency or fellowship positions at the end of your time with them. Be aware and keep track with a paper or electronic grid of how you feel each person is performing on rounds, doing presentations, writing notes, interacting with patients, and showing an appropriate fund of knowledge. If you do not feel you can give an excellent recommendation, say so immediately. Suggest that you are willing to change your mind if his or her performance is upgraded.

At the first attending rounds, in addition to asking what the team wants from you, openly discuss your expectations of them, such as punctuality. Be clear about the time and place you will meet, and for how long, and state that you expect to go to the bedside unless the patient is at a procedure or x-ray.

Go over when the students on the team will be expected to present to you. Let them know that you encourage them to do research on their patients' problems and report back to you and the team what they learn on a daily basis.

Encourage senior residents to be the "faculty member" for one day a week and have them give a five- to ten-minute presentation on a topic of their choice. Finally, set the tone for your expectations that your team will present the cases accurately, deliver outstanding medical care, and have fun and learn a lot. Your enthusiasm about seeing patients and teaching at the bedside is essential to your success. Setting high expectations and goals for your weeks with the team is crucial for excellent patient care to occur. Remember to inquire about the days that your team members will not be at rounds due to clinic assignments. Write down the clinic assignments for each member so that you are not looking for him or her to appear at those times. Having the beeper or cell phone numbers for each person on your team will enable you to contact him or her with questions or concerns.

Earlier attending faculty involvement in inpatient decision making has been shown by Wachter et al. (1998) to improve patient length of stay while not affecting mortality, patient outcomes, or resident satisfaction. Therefore, I ask the resident to call me about each admission that comes in from the emergency room under my name as the attending of record. Seeing the emergency admission the day he or she arrives is far preferable to waiting until the next day, when many decisions about tests and therapeutics will have already been made. You may not agree with what was done without your approval, but it is often too late to reverse the decisions, the direction, and the momentum of the case.

You have two major functions as the attending for an inpatient service, whether it be a medicine, surgery, pediatrics, obstetrics and gynecology service, or any other service—to help make the best possible patient care decisions and to teach house staff and medical students about the disease entity and your decision-making process. As part of your functions, you will be expected to see patients at the bedside, model proper physician-patient interactions, unravel cases, help put a plan together for the resolution of the problem, and teach an evidence-based approach to disease.

Showcase Your Clinical Skills during Attending Rounds

Attending rounds are primarily designed to showcase two skills: (1) the attending physician's problem-solving skills, and (2) the attending physician's communication skills during physician-patient interactions. The attending is expected to provide a thoughtful analysis of the patient's case and of facts put forth during rounds. The higher-order objectives of Bloom's taxonomy (1956) (namely, analysis, synthesis, and evaluation) are optimally displayed while watching the attending and team brainstorm to try to solve a case or make a difficult decision after weighing the pros and cons of the diagnostic and therapeutic modalities available. Many hospitals have developed teams of attendings using one subspecialist and one generalist on a rounding team to give adequate coverage of general medical problems and of specialty knowledge. I take a Socratic approach to solving the mystery case presented, by asking a variety of questions of the team members. This keeps everyone on his or her toes and advances the team as a decision-making body. X-rays and lab data are excellent items to use as focal points for questions to individual team members. What do you think this shows? What is the significance? What would you do next? Why do you say that?

Attending physicians demonstrate communication skills with patients during rounds. They are held to high standards by students and residents who want to learn this complex and difficult skill from an expert. J. Willis Hurst (1999, 37) notes, "A true teacher is a good communicator. True teachers sense when trainees they are teaching understand what they are saying. And they work to be understood."

Bedside Teaching

Excellent teaching requires no magic. Behind-the-scenes preparation is the key to an effective and successful teaching presentation (fig. 8.1). Bedside teaching, while looking like the most unrehearsed activity, is actually the most rehearsed and labor intensive, if it is to go well. Great bedside skills should both impress and be copied by your team members. A study from Australia (Young et al. 2009) that evaluated teaching and learning on clinical rotations turned up the surprising finding that passive and low-level cognitive actions dominated (teacher asks rhetorical or closed question, shares knowledge in a didactic manner), particularly at the bedside. This does not have to be the way bedside teaching is perceived. Crumlish, Yialamas, and McMahon (2009) noted that bedside teaching was responsible for only 17 percent of the time spent teaching by an academic hospitalist group; physical examinations are less frequent than they were in the past. These authors call for strategies to improve bedside teaching and re-emphasize its importance to patient care.

Teaching Success

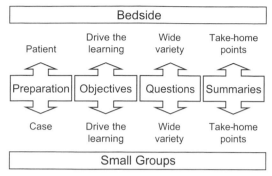

Figure 8.1. **Teaching Successes at the Bedside or in Small Groups Depend on Preparation, Learning Objectives, Questions, and a Final Summary**
Do background reading in preparation for a patient case discussion at the bedside or in a small group. Drive the learning with predetermined objectives and carefully thought-out questions that cover the objectives. Always summarize at the end with useful, bottom-line, take-home points, based on your expertise and evidence from the current literature.

Terrific communication skills are essential for the consummate bedside physician. Levinson et al. (1997) showed that physician-patient communication differed in primary care physicians who had no malpractice claims versus those that did have malpractice claims. The no-claims physicians laughed more, educated patients about what to expect, asked for patients' opinions, and encouraged patients to talk. Put your expert communication skills on display for the team and the patient. Eat and drink coffee, tea, or whatever drink is most energy sustaining for you before you go in to see and talk with a difficult patient. Remember to shake hands with each patient after publicly washing your hands or using the hospital dispenser with antibacterial cleanser, and have your nametag clearly visible. Sit in a chair so that you look into the patient's eyes. Do not look at your team unless you need to communicate with them about ordering tests or you wish to emphasize something the patient has said for their benefit. Explain to the patient that you are eager for the entire team to hear your conversation and ask if this is all right with him or her. Show the patient that you are an advocate while showing the team how to win a patient's trust and confidence.

Prepare by finding out, if possible, the names of the patients to be presented on rounds, their tentative diagnoses, and the questions the house staff have asked the consult services. Alternatively, as the attending, you may choose a patient that you believe will provide an excellent learning experience, and ask that patient if he or she is willing to participate in a bedside teaching exercise. Then, go to the nurse and make sure the patient will be in his or her room during teaching rounds, review the record, and decide what point(s) you wish to make. Your audience at the bedside does not care if you have seen the patient before or rehearsed your presentation, but they do want rounds to be a productive and engaging learning experience, so prepare in the following manner:

1. Visualize yourself teaching and decide on how much time and what points are to be covered in the hall outside the patient's room, at the bedside, and in the conference room. Bedside teaching can include going to the pathology and radiology departments if the slides or x-rays are already pulled and you have enlisted the help of the pathologist or radiologist or to help your team have a good teaching experience. Be organized. The easiest way to get teaching accolades is to conceive a viable and practical teaching plan and then execute it smoothly. House staff and fellows are often too busy to cope with the necessary details for the teaching to occur. To have sufficient time to prepare to teach and to do the teaching, block your schedule appropriately for teaching. Minimize your own outpatient practice hours and procedures during your teaching time.

2. Develop objectives for each day of attending rounds. Let the group know what you plan to teach that day. Decide what open-ended, diagnostic, informational, or clarifying questions you will ask to make your major teaching points.

3. Focus on one or two objectives or teaching points that you wish to make. Restrain your desire to teach everything in one day's session. One or two pearls are sufficient. Vary the emphasis by switching from discussing the pathophysiology of a disease one day, a remarkable history or interesting physical findings another day, to the latest treatment on the next day. Shift the level of your comments from fellow to house staff to student.

4. Plan to give each member of your teaching group a role in the bedside exercise, such as taking the history, examining the abdomen, communicating a finding, or being the observer and describer. Do not

plan to do all of the teaching yourself; it will be less engaging than involving each member of the team over time.

5. Anchor your points using review articles, classic papers, a broad differential diagnosis, or a well-chosen diagram of how to do a certain physical finding.

6. Be confident that you know more than those whom you are teaching. Prepare by reading ahead of time, but feel free to say "I do not know the answer and I will look it up for rounds tomorrow." Remember to write down the question, or you may forget to look up items you promised to research.

7. A wide variety of teaching techniques at the bedside are effective:

   a. Showcase history-taking skills. Important history may be obtained by the attending physician: A patient who has diarrhea is found to be taking senna in an herbal over-the-counter preparation obtained from a health food store.

   b. Demonstrate physical diagnosis skills: Show the method for eliciting costovertebral angle tenderness in a patient whose abdominal pain may be due to pyelonephritis.

   c. Illustrate role-modeling behavior: Go to the bedside of a disgruntled patient and reveal your methods for soothing this patient's anger.

   d. Model culturally competent care: Show how you would work with the patient whose culture may not permit him or her to take a treatment that is essential to improving the illness.

   e. Use questions to stimulate discussion at the bedside: Using open-ended questions such as "What do you think is going on?" or "How would you prioritize the tests you wish to request?" may lead to a vibrant discussion.

   f. Deliver a five-minute minilecture at the bedside: If the patient has ascites, consider giving the definition, microbiology, predisposing factors, diagnosis, and treatment of spontaneous bacterial peritonitis while examining the patient at the bedside.

   g. Observe and give feedback: Be frank with praise for histories and physical exams well done but correct immediately any improperly taken histories and physical exams. Gentle correction, minus personal attack, is the key to learning without embarrassing the learner.

8. Signatures, notes, and other housekeeping details should be accomplished after teaching rounds have been completed.

9. Even if only one student, house staff member, or resident shows up at the bedside because other duties or emergencies have sidelined the rest of the group, forge ahead with your teaching presentation. Do not wait for the ideal time when the entire group is together. It may never occur, and it is disrespectful to the lone but eager learner who did show up. If the lone learner gives good feedback about your presentation that the others missed, more will come to the next sessions.

Experience Counts

Sometimes you feel that the residents and fellows know more of the latest literature than you do. You wonder what you can teach them. The team, on the other hand, aspires to gain from your experience and your approach to diagnosis and management. They frequently recognize that you may not quote the latest journal article or provide evidence-based medical studies off the tip of your tongue. They are often better than you are at rapid recall. But, you have numerous complex cases under your belt and grateful patients to prove your successful treatment. Use your experience-based wisdom to teach your team salient points about history, physical diagnosis, x-ray interpretation, and interactions with the nurses and ward secretaries and staff. Make points about politics, insurance, free care, medication counselors to obtain free medications for the financially needy patient, and about how to engage the difficult patient or the frightened or depressed patient in a fruitful dialogue.

Orchestrate a memorable patient interaction at a bedside after you have interviewed the patient carefully and obtained his or her permission to be interviewed in bed, in the solarium or patient lounge, or with family. This memorable event may be far more important to the resident struggling to know what to say and how to handle certain situations than a discussion of the merits and weaknesses of the latest clinical or research study.

Reflect on what makes you special as a physician, and teach this skill to your team. Patients have told you over the years what they like about your style in the office or on the phone or in your interactions with their families. Try to bottle these special qualities by naming them to yourself. Are you responsive, caring, kind, patient, resourceful, an advocate, brilliant as a diagnostician, terrific with your hands? Do you perform a thorough physical exam, have great listening ability, understanding, and comprehension of social or economic issues? On rounds, go to great lengths to show the qualities you and your patients are proud of. These are worthwhile to try to transmit during teaching rounds. However, you must specifically plan ahead of time to try to show these excellent traits to both the patient and the team so that the residents, fellows, students, pharmacy interns, and nurses can watch you in action and remember how complex situations can be handled with finesse. Do not hesitate to name for the team the qualities that have endeared you to a difficult patient population. All physicians want to be successful, but few achieve uniform success at the bedside unless they work hard to mold their behavior to be soothing and reassuring. Some physicians have a gift for making patients feel better just by shaking hands with them and meeting their gaze. This useful skill can be cultivated.

Residents and fellows want cases for their weekly teaching conferences and for publication (Teunissen and Dornan 2008). Watch out for great cases that you and your team see that are publishable, with you as senior author and the resident/fellow or student as first author. Nothing endears you more to the team than your helping them to succeed by lengthening their bibliography through supervising their writing up of cases.

Mechanics

At the beginning of rounds, on a daily basis, outline when time for teaching will be occurring and tell the team what you expect to do. Are you giving a "chalk talk," going over interesting x-rays, giving a canned slide talk, leading them to the bedside of a patient with an interesting finding, or having your team review a mystery case that teaches an important point? If you have prepared a teaching moment or talk, do not ask your team on that day what they wish to hear from you or you may be derailed from what you are ready to teach. On the other hand, if multiple emergencies occur during rounds or a code is called on one of the team's patients, it is best to drop plans for specific teaching and focus on helping the team think through the difficult decisions they face on one or more patients that day, even if these are not your patients.

If you have had a fellow or resident on service before, he or she may have already heard your canned talk, mystery case, or "chalk talk." Ask the resident or fellow if he or she has heard the talk before. If so, suggest another topic you can discuss or ask if he or she would like to hear this talk again. Whatever the topic, make it an interactive session by asking questions as you move through your material, getting plenty of input from the team. Adult learners want to be involved and to participate. Give them every opportunity by asking questions or posing problems for them to solve, such as minivignettes with one remarkable x-ray or pathologic finding.

Have one or all of the senior residents and students give a talk, if they wish, on a topic of interest to them and the team. Give him or her feedback after the presentation on how it went from your point of view and what changes, if any, you would suggest for the next time.

Find Teachable Moments

Do not wait for a set-aside time to teach. Make each attending round a teachable moment by delivering a running commentary out loud on why you are doing something the way you are doing it. Confer with your team about what you are planning to say or do in each patient's room before you go in, and then discuss with them what they thought of the physician-patient interaction when you come out of the room.

If you plan to do bedside teaching, ask the patient ahead of time if it is all right with him or her to teach at the bedside. Although patients are usually happy for the opportunity to listen to a discussion of their case, it is possible that they will not appreciate this, and you must respect their wishes.

For those in training to learn proper bedside skills, it is worthwhile to deconstruct for them what they are seeing. They may be seeing one thing and you and other team members other things. It is often good to ask "So, what happened in there?" and hear the variety of responses from the hierarchy of team members (fellows, residents, students, pharmacy or nursing interns, nurses, nurse's assistants, social workers), listing and then analyzing what each person saw (similar to the 1950 film *Rashomon,* by the director Akira Kurasawa).

It is never too late to become a great teacher on rounds. Know your strengths and play to them. Before joining you for their first rounds, the group you are working with will have gone over your strengths and weaknesses with others who know your teaching style. Given the advance publicity, play to your strengths and minimize your weaknesses. Remember the negative and positive evaluations you have received over the years, and try to avoid falling into negative traps that have ensnared you in the past and led to your receiving mediocre or even poor ratings. The team will be pleasantly surprised that you are not running true to form.

Team members do not want you to waste their time. Watching you write a note is not a valuable learning experience unless you consult them about the wording of a particularly complex patient note, which may be sent to a several other consultants. You should write your notes, unless they are emergencies, on your own time, after rounds are have been completed. An interested student or resident may wish to see how you phrase things, but it is best to declare rounds over and let the team members accomplish their own important patient-care tasks that rounds have kept them from.

Be careful of playing favorites. This is especially true when students or residents state that they wish to go into the specialty you are in. Often, you will focus more attention on them. Pleasing these students or residents or keeping them interested suddenly becomes paramount. However, the rest of the team will become restless, frustrated, and disenchanted if this lopsided focus persists.

Respect the hierarchy. Do not show up the fellow in front of the senior resident or the junior resident in front of the student. A junior member may outshine a more senior member of the team in differential diagnosis. Remedy this by asking each person to alternate in guessing the answer. Then the more senior member, who may be slower on the draw, has the opportunity to show that he or she knows the answers well but is not as quick to name the abnormality in a competitive situation.

Have your idea of how rounds will go, but consult the senior member of the team beforehand to make sure that he or she did not have other ideas on how the rounds should function.

It may turn out that several members of your team have afternoon clinics and that rounds that afternoon will begin at 5 p.m., after a long clinic session for both residents. You may make early rounds with the team and come back on your own to work with the medical students in the afternoon, when the residents are in clinic. To avoid delaying your input on consults, you may have had only one team member with you when you saw patients earlier in the day. It may then be best to regroup for a day's summary at 5 p.m., in the cafeteria with snacks or with coffee at the chart rack and computers, to discuss the patients who are very ill and check on their data. Evening rounds with your team will focus on new consults waiting to be seen, viewing x-rays with attending radiologists before telling the patients the results, and rounding on sick patients together as a team to formulate the plan for that evening and the next day.

Always be respectful of the patient, even if your team is not. Model the proper behavior to the younger physicians, who sometimes let their feelings about the patient "hang out." Their having negative feelings about a particular patient may be warranted, but letting the patient see them is not a therapeutic maneuver unless the patient is an alcoholic or a substance abuse patient who is unwilling to follow hospital rules and poses a risk to him- or herself and to other patients or staff.

Assessment with a Miniclinical Evaluation Exercise

The American Board of Internal Medicine (ABIM) recommends that program directors employ a bedside oral examination for evaluating first-year residents (Norcini et al. 2003). Originally, the Clinical Evaluation Exercise (CEX) had the faculty member watching the resident perform a complete history and physical examination on one of the inpatients and evaluating the quality of both the history and the physical exam, as well as the diagnostic and therapeutic conclusions—a process that took approximately two hours (Norcini et al. 1995). In response to criticisms of the CEX being a single assessment by one examiner with differences in grading, the ABIM changed its recommendation to the Mini-CEX. In the Mini-CEX, one faculty member observes a first-year resident during fifteen- to twenty-minute encounters with patients (Norcini et al. 1995). Several encounters are observed by different faculty members in the course of the year and in different settings, such as the emergency room, an outpatient setting, and an inpatient setting, so that the resident can demonstrate skills in a broader array of patients. The mini-CEX requires the resident to show his or her ability to focus and prioritize the diagnosis and management plans for patients in a real clinical-practice setting. Norcini et al. (2003) showed that when 21 sites and 421 residents were evaluated using a standard rating form during each of the four quarters of the year, the residents' skills significantly improved over the year. Skills were highest for professionalism and lowest for physical examination. They concluded that the Mini-CEX, while not having the resident observed over the course of an entire history and physical exam, did provide for several different faculty members to observe a broader sample of residents' skills, with a wide variety of patient problems in a range of settings.

Feedback

A crucial component of the teaching-attending physician's job is the evaluation of residents and the assessment of whether they are capable of practicing independently (Holmboe 2004; Kogan, Holmboe, and Hauer 2009; Steinmann et al. 2009). Kogan, Holmboe, and Hauer (2009) noted that direct observation of medical trainees by teaching faculty remains an important component of assessment for medical educators. Dorfsman and Wolfson (2009) reported that a new direct observation program was well received by Emergency Department second-year residents and gave the faculty insights into the strengths and weaknesses of both individuals and the group. Beaumier et al. (1992) reported on the difficulties most frequently encountered among first-year family medicine residents. Incomplete history taking was the number one problem, followed by improper physical examination technique.

Teaching faculty need to give detailed assessment and feedback to trainees to prepare them to practice at the highest levels of clinical competence. Take team members aside for feedback, positive or negative, on a weekly basis. Try to give the feedback immediately, when the positive or negative interaction or case presentation occurs. Feedback is much more memorable when given in relation to an event that can still be well remembered. Learn to praise and to constructively criticize a team member as the work is done. Do not to store up negative feelings but offer observations on patients well or poorly cared for promptly. Ask the team member how he or she felt about the performance or decision making. Often this is the opening the person is looking for to discuss disappointment with his or her own clinical judgment or skills. Dispassionate criticisms will sink in better, and you will give the person a chance to correct a pattern of shoddy care, a lack of follow-through, inadequate background knowledge, a brusque way of speaking, or carelessness about data collection or note writing then and there. The student may still have time to show that he or she can improve and gain your respect for his or her skills. If immediate feedback is difficult to give, then have a set time during the week to discuss any opinion, evaluations, or tentative grades you would give to members of the team. Ask them at least weekly how rounds are going and what they would like to do differently the next time. Ask frankly how you are doing as a teacher and as a ward attending. If no criticisms are given and no changes are suggested, ask again on a weekly basis. See Chapter 6 for additional tips on feedback.

Reflections and Refinement

Actualization is doing rounds with the fellows, residents, or team. Reflect on what you did and how it went in order to improve your performance (refinement). Listen to the nagging voice that says things were not as smooth as you wished or did not seem to result in openness and eagerness. Listen to the voice that says the patient had a good time, but the residents and interns seemed edgy and bored.

Changing how you do something in teaching medicine is not easy for someone who has been teaching for years and is proud of his or her track record. However, each learner group is different. What one group liked last year may not be what your current group likes. Be sure to recognize that the path to bad evaluations is paved by not paying attention or by ignoring the telltale signs that your actions and words are not appreciated. Unless you intervene quickly, those negative evaluations about your sensitivity, knowledge base, feedback to the group, tardiness for rounds, or excessively long rounds will be put into your permanent teaching folder.

Inpatient Specialty Attending Physician

Specialty fellows and residents expect slightly different teaching from the designated attending physician compared to the general medicine and surgery residents. Specialists want to learn both the basics and the nuances of the diagnosis, management, and therapeutics for the particular common and uncommon diseases of the specialty. Your years of practice and success are appealing to your recruits and those who wish to emulate you. Fellows particularly want to know when and how to perform procedures, when complications may occur, and what to do about them. The specialist resident or fellow is more motivated to want your opinion and to watch you interact with the patient to see excellent communication skills in action. Because their training is soon to be over, fellows are generally apt learners. Because they will soon be attendings, they recognize that they need a certain body of knowledge for this role, as well as a certain style, to be successful.

Outpatient Teaching
Complex Schedules Need Forethought

Far more complicated than making inpatient rounds, in a controlled setting where the cases are discussed relatively leisurely and the patient is brought into the discussion at a prescribed time, is teaching in the ambulatory setting. Aagaard, Teherani, and Irby (2004, 42) noted that "teachers . . . struggle to find ways to integrate students into their busy practices while minimizing the disruption to patient care." As only the sickest patients are admitted to inpatient wards, most patients have their diagnostic and therapeutic decisions made in the outpatient arena. Both third-year students and residents now spend considerable time in outpatient areas and require supervised teaching. The difficulties for the teacher are how to maintain excellent patient care and continuity while having students independently see patients and be supervised on their findings and plans and yet not drop their productivity and billing too much. Weinberger, Smith, and Collier (2006) state that ambulatory experiences in internal medicine programs are a lower priority than the inpatient service and are often not well designed.

Dent and Hesketh (2003) proposed multiple educational models, along with their advantages and disadvantages, for medical students to see outpatients with supervision, including grandstanding, in which the student observes the tutor; breakout, in which the student observes initially and then interviews the patient individually; supervising, in which the student practices history and physical exam with supervision; and report back, in which a senior student examines a patient independently and reports the findings to the faculty member. Faculty need to prepare and have a plan for which model he or she is choosing before arriving in the clinic. Irby et al. (1991) found that nurturing autonomy and self-directed learning were key factors in successful teaching in the outpatient setting.

Lesky and Hershman (1995) note that smooth functioning of an outpatient area requires adequate examination room space, a student-preceptor schedule that maximizes efficiency and teaching time, a system for informing patients and obtaining their consent, a plan for orienting students to the clinic environment and the support staff, and a discrete space for the learner to read and write notes and for teaching to occur without standing and talking in the hallway. Revenues will be less when teaching takes place in the outpatient area.

However, Lesky and Hershman (1995) propose several teaching and scheduling strategies that decrease the impact of the losses. Residents and students need a private exam room to see patients but do not need it for the entire time of the clinic—only for the purpose of the history and physical exam. Therefore, the preceptor and the student or resident can share two exam rooms, and the student can do all tasks that do not require an exam room in a work room or library where there is computer access. Lesky and Hershman (1995) suggest a schedule in which the preceptor and student see patients at the same time, but the next slot for the preceptor is held open for supervision and teaching of the student about his or her patient. This design maintains the same number of patients seen by the preceptor for a session and minimizes wasted time, permitting a maximum amount for time for teaching.

I notify patients before a clinic when I will have students, residents, or fellows, even if the learner is shadowing rather than seeing the patient independently. Patients who are seen by the student will generally be delayed for twenty to thirty minutes owing to the teaching by the preceptor and being seen by resident, fellow, or student and the preceptor. Clinic staff should be informed of the student's arrival and the student's name and year of training. The staff can be extremely helpful to the student who is learning the ropes of the clinic and the laboratory.

Setting the Stage for a Successful Experience

When a student, resident, or fellow first comes into your clinic:

1. Find out the areas in which these learners think that they need more knowledge or experience.
2. Figure out these areas by going over each learner's previous outpatient rotations and specialty clinics.
3. Work with the learners on topics of particular interest to them.
4. Ask about what they perceive as possible knowledge gaps in their history-taking skills or physical examinations.
5. Compile a list of illnesses commonly seen in your office and have the learners choose those to which they would like greater exposure.
6. Plan the work schedule together, including which patients are excellent for them to see, what articles they should read, and the names of other physicians who may help them learn the areas in which they feel deficient.

7. Educational objectives in the outpatient setting are generally put into one of three domains of learning: the cognitive domain, which deals with the recall or recognition of factual knowledge; the affective domain, with focuses on verbal skills, language, attitudes, and values; and the psychomotor domain, which refers to objectives related to procedural skills. Find out what objectives are of greatest interest to your learners.

8. Explain how feedback will be given.

9. Ask what their long-term career goals are.

10. Ask how they wish to be introduced to patients.

11. Describe your style for teaching and precepting in the outpatient area.

The Five-Step Microskills, or One-Minute Preceptor Model

Aagaard, Teherani, and Irby (2004) compared Neher et al.'s (1992) Five-Step Microskills method, subsequently called the One-Minute Preceptor, with traditional models of ambulatory teaching. Preceptors viewed scripted, videotaped teaching encounters, using the One-Minute Preceptor model developed by Jon Neher and colleagues (1992), in the Department of Family Medicine at the University of Washington, in Seattle, for efficient and effective outpatient teaching of residents. This One-Minute Preceptor model is learner-centered, unlike a traditional patient-centered model, and it was rated as more efficient and effective. The traditional ambulatory teaching model focuses on:

- Listening to the case presentation by the student
- Questioning the student about the data
- Discussing the case and plan for patient care

Little teaching and feedback occur in the traditional model, in which the preceptor is functioning as an expert consultant who is trying to pick up on areas missed by the learner and on the learner's understanding of the preceptor's plan for the patient.

The Five-Step Microskills, or One-Minute Preceptor, model encourages the preceptor to do the following:

1. Obtain a commitment from the learner about what he or she thinks is wrong with the patient.

2. Question the reasoning by probing for supporting evidence.

3. Provide general rules of clinical medicine or salient take-home points.
4. Give positive feedback, reinforcing what was done right.
5. Correct mistakes in thinking, diagnosis, or management.

Each of these five steps is elaborated on below.

Obtain a Commitment

If the resident or student makes a commitment to a diagnosis or plan of action, he or she will usually feel more responsible for the patient's care and be more involved in solving the problem at hand. Asking for a commitment forces the resident to analyze the data collected during the history and physical exam and encourages the learner to make sense of it then and there. The preceptor should use this skill when the learner has presented the facts of the case. When the presentation is finished, the learner awaits the preceptor's comments. Instead of commenting, the preceptor should ask the learner what he or she thinks about the data just presented with a simple open-ended question such as "What do you think is going on?" or "What tests would you like to order?" The preceptor should limit questions that ask for additional data to a few key items. The focus at this point should be on the learner's problem-solving capabilities.

Probe for Supporting Evidence

After the learner has made a commitment to a diagnosis and a plan, the preceptor should try to elucidate the thought processes that led the learner to this decision. Because the learner's diagnosis is derived from the data collected, this step permits preceptor and learner to identify what the learner knows and does not know. The learner will ask the preceptor for confirmation of the diagnosis. Here the preceptor should ask for the evidence that supports the diagnosis with a question such as "What facts led you to that conclusion?"

Teach General Rules

If the learner's reasoning is correct, then there may be little to teach. However, if there are deficiencies in how the case was put together or analyzed, then the preceptor should offer some general rules of clinical medicine. Avoid anecdotes and make the teaching points succinct and broad. For example, "If the patient has bright red blood per rectum and is over age 50, a colonoscopy should be performed to ascertain the source of bleeding and to screen for colon polyps and colon cancer."

Reinforce What Was Done Right

Give the learner a specific example of what he or she did well. If the patient is jaundiced, the resident should be praised for percussing the liver and measuring the size to be 18 cm in the right midclavicular line and for ascertaining that asterixis is present. This praise will act as reinforcement for doing a competent targeted physical exam, focusing on answering several questions that flow logically from having noted jaundice.

Correct Mistakes

Neher et al. (1992) note that correcting mistakes requires tact and a sense of timing for when to give negative feedback. Although best done close to the event, it may have to be delayed for a private time, which permits freer conversation than the busy clinic. The preceptor's prime focus should be not only on correcting the mistake but also on avoiding it in the future. The mistake may be labeled as "not best practice" rather than "bad" practice. An example of this type of feedback might be as follows: "When a patient comes in with a history of a black tarry stool, it is essential to check the patient's stool with a fecal occult blood card to verify that there is actually blood in the stool. Products that contain iron or bismuth can lead to a black stool, too. Please do a rectal exam and check the stool for blood next time before jumping to the conclusion that the patient has a gastrointestinal bleed, when instead, iron is the culprit." Avoid being vague or judgmental. The five-step microskills model is perfect for a specialty clinic as well.

Other methods for organizing the outpatient-teaching visit are *priming* and *framing*. With the priming technique, the attending gives the learner pertinent background information on the patient problem just before he or she sees the patient. The attending also asks the student or resident specific questions about the symptoms, the physical findings that he or she may find during the visit with the patient. Priming helps guide the learner's history and physical exam in a focused manner.

Framing sets expectations and parameters for what the attending expects the learner to accomplish and also sets time limits. It helps increase the efficiency of the learner's outpatient experience by encouraging him or her to accomplish a focused task, such as working up gnawing upper abdominal pain with a targeted history, and a focused physical exam within fifteen to twenty minutes and then reporting back to the attending with the findings.

✒ TEACHING TIPS

1. Create good will early; make inpatient rounds interesting, fun, and informative.
2. Balance your patients' needs with your learners' needs; this delicate and important balance is the key to success.
3. Clear the decks of deadlines, papers, manuscripts, and grant applications; focus on being intellectually and physically ready.
4. Clearly articulate your expectations for your clinical team members early in your attending block; set up the right dynamic.
5. Do not wait for the right time to teach; house staff may be called away.
6. Focus on one or two objectives each day, and vary the emphasis; variety is the spice of life.
7. Use your experience to teach salient points of history, physical diagnosis, and cross-cultural care.
8. Notify patients that a resident or student may be seeing them in your clinic; give each patient the opportunity to say no.
9. Use the One-Minute Preceptor model for outpatient teaching; it will pay off.
10. Increase efficiency and focused learning in the outpatient arena by using *priming* and *framing,* two excellent alternative attending teaching techniques.

✒ TAKE-HOME POINTS

- Clinical attending teaching duties require time and effort. Block your schedule accordingly.
- Rehearse and prepare behind the scenes to make bedside rounds go smoothly as a teaching exercise.
- Create a comfortable learning environment.
- Give prepared minitalks on common subjects.
- Showcase your problem-solving skills and your communication skills with patients during inpatient rounds and outpatient clinics.
- Make the outpatient clinic experience helpful for learners by probing the reasoning and focusing on the problem-solving capabilities of each learner.

CHAPTER NINE

Postgraduate Teaching

- *What are the hallmarks of an excellent postgraduate lecture?*
- *How do I prepare and deliver a great grand-rounds presentation?*
- *Is small-group learning similar to problem-based learning?*
- *What preparations are necessary for problem-based learning at the postgraduate level?*
- *What do workshop participants want?*
- *What are the duties of a course director?*
- *How do I prepare to be a moderator at a national meeting?*
- *What are the keys to a poster presentation?*
- *How do I give a flawless platform presentation at a national meeting?*

Expectations of Postgraduate Learning

Postgraduate audiences expect value for the time away from their offices and the money they spend to attend the session. Polished, professional presentations using strong organizational and audiovisual skills are essential to getting concepts across. Teaching others at the local or national level for credit means enhancing learning over and above what is offered locally. This requires a thorough knowledge of the subject to pitch the learning at the correct level. Participants who have paid for the session will be upset if the knowledge transmitted is at a low level and frustrated if it at a level over their heads. The postgraduate teacher should know the expectations of the specialty boards to focus the presentation on classic and time-honored concepts as well as to bring in new data, innovations, and controversial, but important, areas. Evidence from the literature is needed to support each recommendation, and a well-researched bibliography is mandatory.

Lecture Presentations

One of the more frustrating things I have witnessed is a graduate medical education lecture, grand rounds, or visiting professor lecture that fails because of technical difficulties (Sands and McGee 2001, http://Home.caregroup.org/

clinical/docs/presenting_your_work.doc). To avoid this, I have assembled a list of questions for you to ask yourself before each major presentation so that you recognize the numerous ways in which your presentation can be ruined despite your hard work (table 9.1).

Smoothly Managing the Technical Part of Your Presentation

Think of your potential technical problems from the beginning because they could be your worst nightmare. After all the preparation, your slides may not be compatible with the system and will not project with the equipment available. Another nightmare is the liquid crystal display (LCD) projector malfunctioning. If it is an important lecture, I recommend the following arduous, but essential, steps to avoid a fiasco.

1. Send a copy of your talk by e-mail or CD ahead of time to the person sponsoring your talk. Be sure to alert his or her administrator. Wait to hear that he or she has received it. Ask the administrator to test it on the system to be sure that animations or video clips will project smoothly. Certain brands of memory stick may be incompatible with the computer system being used. Check ahead to see if this is an issue.
2. Consider bringing your own laptop and check that it will show your slides and video clips as a backup.
3. Bring your own LCD projector, which is compatible with your laptop.
4. Send your slide presentation ahead so that it can be printed out and photocopied for each audience member, with page numbers.
5. Check whether the Continuing Medical Education office expects you to hand out copies of your lecture notes. If so, send them your lecture note file.
6. When in doubt, delete animations and video clips that may not be able to be shown. Focus on giving an excellent talk without glitches.
7. Write out your talk on index cards or have a typed copy so that if the slides will not project, you will still get your major message across.
8. Check out the lighting ahead of time to decide what level is needed for your talk. Make sure you can see the audience to watch their response to your lecture. This gives you valuable feedback. If the body language of the audience is not enthusiastic or positive, try to adjust your talk on the spot to improve your delivery. Consider asking the audience a question to get them more engaged.

Table 9.1.   Technical Questions to Ask before a Presentation

1. What if my slide presentation is not compatible with the computer and projector system where I am presenting?
2. Will there be media experts to help me load my presentation ahead of time?
3. Should I e-mail or send a CD of my presentation to the moderator or my contact and ask him or her to load it on the computer and check that it will open properly?
4. How early should I arrive at the auditorium before my presentation?
5. Should I bring my own laptop computer?
6. Should I bring a liquid crystal display projector? Should I bring an extra light bulb?
7. How do I find out the name of the person who will be helping me with my presentation?
8. How much of my reputation is riding on this single lecture?
9. How much will my reputation suffer if my talk does not go well?
10. How much will it help my career if the talk goes extremely well?
11. Are there old friends or former mentors in the audience?
12. Should I bring hard copies of everything?
13. Do I trust that my contacts and their administrators will have copies of my slides ready for handout for a grand rounds presentation if I send them my slide set?
14. Will they paginate the slides' pages so that, if my slide show fails, I can refer to the slide and page number?
15. Am I trying to teach something interesting or am I just trying to show the overwhelming number of beautiful slides I have?
16. Am I going to leave any room for questions?

Making up Slides

1. Less is more. Allow one minute for most word slides, one and a half minutes for charts and table explanations, and thirty seconds for describing photographs of histology, pathology, endoscopy, surgical specimens, or x-rays.
2. Use only one line for each bullet point, if possible.
3. Make up slides with a limit of six words per line.
4. Stick to only four to six points per slide.
5. Use a large enough font for the slide to be easily read in the back of the room (24–36 point).
6. Add variety by using photos, tables, graphics, or diagrams rather than just plain text for each slide.
7. Avoid crowding the slide with information.
8. Make the title for each slide both simple and direct.

9. Reference carefully all data slides, illustrations, and quotes and put the reference on the slide using the author's last name, the journal, year, volume, and page numbers.

10. Design colorful slides and an attractive talk.

11. Spend time getting the best photograph or diagram.

12. Avoid dense tables. If you must show a table, use a highlighter to direct attention toward the line you wish to discuss.

13. If your lecture is sixty minutes, then forty slides is a maximum. This will leave you with little time for questions, however.

14. If your lecture is twenty minutes, fourteen slides are sufficient.

15. Slides should be clear and uncluttered, with large legible font (e.g., Times New Roman, Courier, Modern, Arial, or Century). The slide title is generally 36 point while the main text is 24 point. The background should be dark blue or black, with white or yellow lettering. Use a red background sparingly.

16. Consider having a uniform color background for your slides even if there are tables and figures.

17. Transitions describe how a slide is brought onto the screen. Images can come from either side or fade in or out. To avoid distracting the audience, stick with one type of transition. Recognize that transitions may slow your presentation and may be annoying for note takers because the slide points appear one by one.

18. Blank slides are helpful when you want the audience to focus on you and your message or as a segue to a new topic.

19. Carefully think out timed slides, where the slide disappears after a set interval. Check before your presentation that the timing is working and that your estimate is correct.

20. Graphic images should each carry a key point and not be decorative.

21. Do not overload slides with information. Long tables and complex meta-analyses should be syllabus material and not be shown during a lecture unless they have been distilled into a word slide. Never apologize for a crowded slide; don't show it.

22. For tables, use only subsets of the data that bring out your key points. Highlight them rather than the entire table sets of data.

Staying within the Time Allotted

Lecturers frequently rush through excessive slide material like a speeding train (Winston 2007a). Many lecturers will delete slides during the lecture as they realize that they will not finish on time. This sets the audience on edge as they wonder what crucial content they have missed, and they downgrade the lecturer for not having done the chore of choosing which slides to show ahead of time. The audience gets the message from the rushed speaker that he or she did not practice the talk for the time allotted. The suspicion of a canned talk, made for another occasion, begins to creep in.

The time to do the selective deleting is in the privacy of your office or home. Take the time carefully and thoughtfully to assort the slides and delete any that are not essential. Give a clear, focused, and relaxed message. Remember that, no matter how important or famous you are, your audience has other pressing things to do once your time is up. They will not stay to hear you but will leave while you are still talking. This unpleasant thought should motivate you to throw out some favorite slides to complete your lecture, on time, with a short, clear summary of important points.

Making Your Lecture Professional

1. Practice your talk out loud, preferably with a projector.
2. Stand up to simulate the real speech.
3. Use a pointer in advance of a major lecture to highlight points on your slides.
4. If you have a shaky hand under the stress of speaking, you may wish to minimize pointing because the tremor can be a distraction. Note where the item of interest is on a slide (e.g., in the right upper corner) as you are speaking. Alternatively, remake the slide with an arrow pointing to the item of interest.
5. Time yourself, making sure you get through your whole talk at least once in the allotted time.
6. Recognize how long your talk will take without interruptions from questions.
7. Decide if you wish to ask the audience to hold questions until the end. I do not recommend doing this because it can create ill will early in a lecture. An engaged audience enjoys asking questions as they come up.

8. Speak out loud to a mirror or tape your lecture and listen to it.
9. Ask a friend to listen to part or all of the lecture. Take all suggestions without becoming defensive, write them down, and decide later, when you have calmed down, which ones make the most sense for your lecture to succeed. The best suggestions sometimes come from nonmedical interested friends, relatives, and spouses, who want you to succeed, not to fail. Their comments may reflect what they see as a lack of clarity, not staying on target, or a boring delivery.
10. Ask a media expert to review your slides to see which ones make the most impact. Even though the media specialist will not know the nuances of science, he or she will know which slides are easiest to grasp.
11. Remove slides your medical or nonmedical audience finds too complex. I have never regretted omitting a complex slide, but I have many regrets about leaving in slides that were complex, took valuable time away from my major lecture objectives, and left the audience confused (Winston 2007b).

Keeping the Audience Interested and Relaxed

Start on time even if only a few people are there. The start time may not be up to you, but if you are asked, always prefer to start at the given time. Your end time will not be extended. Starting late only puts you behind from the beginning and causes the "rush to catch up" phenomenon.

1. Begin with an engaging story and visual. Win over the audience with your relaxed but enthusiastic manner. The combination of excellent content and showmanship makes for an ideal lecture, as evidenced by studies showing that the expressiveness and enthusiasm of the lecturer can stimulate learning even when the lecturer is actually an actor and has no specific knowledge of the lecture subject (Naftulin, Ware, and Donnelly 1973; Whitman and Schwenk 1997).
2. Look around the auditorium before you begin in order to minimize the jitters when you stand up at the podium. Arrive early enough to observe where you will stand and who is present. Practice how you will sweep the audience with your gaze once you are at the podium.
3. Focus on being engaging; your preparation should permit you to relax and smile.

4. Vary your tone of voice.
5. Be polite and grateful that you have been asked to present.
6. Make your visual aids memorable.
7. Never put anything on a slide or say anything that could be offensive to anyone in the audience, including those of a different gender, race, ethnicity, political party, or socioeconomic status.

Structuring the Lecture

The audience is at your lecture to learn; therefore, teach them logically and clearly (Winston 2007a, 2007b; Westberg and Jason 1991). Outline your goals for yourself and for the audience early on (McLaughlin and Mandin 2001). What do you want them to take away from your talk? Is this a survey lecture, a board review lecture, a research presentation, an update, or a talk explaining a complex concept? Tell them your approach to the material, your lecture plan.

1. Each lecture should have an introduction, a body, and a conclusion.
2. Include, immediately after your title slide, a disclosure slide, outlining any potential conflicts of interest: ties to industry, speakers' bureau, grant support and funding, and board memberships.
3. Announce what you will discuss and what your objectives are. Having and sharing objectives is an Accreditation Council for Graduate Medical Education (ACGME) requirement. Announce your objectives on your first or second slide; stick to no more than four or five points.
4. If you do not wish to put your objectives on a slide, you can say them directly to the audience. In this case, limit the objectives to three, so the audience can more easily remember your lecture plan.
5. Attempt to explain no more than five major points or concepts. Make sure that your objectives match one on one with your content.
6. Explain your key areas one at a time. Limit your content with careful selection; do not try to cover the entire subject.
7. Use clinical material as illustrations, examples, and elaborations.
8. Order your material in the logical sequence.
9. Carefully construct segues between your different points.
10. Reiterate and review each of your points as you go along.
11. Summarize at the end, making sure to touch on each of the key areas (objectives) you have highlighted in your lecture.

Making Your Lecture More Interactive

1. Consider asking questions of the audience. Have many of you have seen this condition? What treatment works best? Ask for their opinions regarding a particular point. Poll them. Make sure you have built in the time for this activity during your lecture. It is not a spur-of-the-moment exercise, but one that has been calculated and well thought out ahead of time.

2. Check with your media services and camera operator, if your lecture is being videotaped, whether you are permitted to move around the auditorium, stage, and aisles, asking for comments or questions. If you can move around, I recommend it as a way of better engaging the audience and maintaining a high level of energy throughout the lecture.

3. Have members of the lecture hall pause, turn to each other (buzz groups) to discuss a controversial point, or share their experiences with what you have been discussing.

4. Use the audience-response system, the scratch card method, or the hand-raising method for recording answers. Sometimes, well-placed questions can give the lecturer and the audience a sense of what is not understood. Create teams as in team-based learning, from different geographic areas of the auditorium, and give out scratch tickets. The scratch ticket answers can be pooled for a team. The different teams' answers can be shouted out to alert you to problems in the audience's understanding. Asking the audience to raise hands can also quickly confirm that something is, or is not, clear.

5. Thank your audience at the end for their attention and participation.

6. Acknowledge all questions asked as "excellent," "probing," "penetrating," "thoughtful," "challenging" "interesting," or "on target."

7. Tell the audience you will stay in the auditorium to answer more questions from those who wish to come up after the lecture is over. Never make your schedule so tight that you must leave the auditorium immediately; this frustrates those who wish to ask a question privately.

Grand Rounds

To be asked to give medical or surgical grand rounds is an honor indicating that you are at the top of your field as a clinician, researcher, or educator. Requests for speakers are made one year in advance. You may be given a topic or asked to suggest a topic. You hope to be asked back again someday. How do you approach giving excellent grand rounds?

1. Know the history of grand rounds as a teaching exercise. Grand rounds has evolved from being a bedside teaching session organized by William Osler (1901) early in the twentieth century and described by him as the "natural method to teach medicine," to a discussion of a patient's illness with the case presentation in the middle of the twentieth century, to being a didactic lecture by the 1980s, sometimes with little clinical relevance or recognition of the audience's needs (Hebert and Wright 2003). Mueller and colleagues at the Mayo Clinic (2006) surveyed ninety-nine departments of medicine regarding medical grand rounds and found that the most common format was a didactic lecture, with no patient and no case presentation. Yet 81 percent of respondents said providing updates in the diagnosis and treatment of disease was the most important objective of grand rounds. Mueller's survey answers led to the following recommendations to improve the quality of grand rounds: (a) protected time to attend, (b) case-based presentations, (c) better audiovisuals, (d) better presenters, (e) facilitation of audience participation, (f) knowledge assessment during or after, with audience response or other methodology, and (g) free food, which is permitted in the auditorium. In addition, enhancing publicity of the grand rounds speaker and topic and conducting yearly surveys of what topics were of educational interest improved grand rounds attendance (Mueller et al. 2003).

2. Understand what grand rounds attendees want. Competing commitments frequently make attending grand rounds difficult. If attendees manage to slip away from clinical and research responsibilities, they want new, evidence-based knowledge regarding clinical or research problems. They also want to obtain a framework for how to approach a particular clinical problem or research breakthrough. Two studies have shown that surgical residents can change behaviors (Reed et al.

2008) and that medical residents acquire knowledge as measured by improved performance on Internal Medicine In-Training Examinations through a one-hour lecture (McDonald, Zeger, and Kolars 2008). At grand rounds, the audience will be diverse. Although composed primarily of general medicine faculty, residents, and students, subspecialty faculty and fellows will also be present. You need to pitch your talk to the faculty level but know what level of knowledge the residents and fellows are expected to have. Glean their knowledge base from their board review books and core curriculum requirements as you research your topic. Do careful literature reviews. Avoid making bold pronouncements during grand rounds unless they are based on current evidence-based studies (Linthorst, Daniels, and Westerloo 2007).

3. Make your objectives clear. Provide impeccable organization to achieve your goal of educating the audience. Make your sequence between key points and within key points a logical progression. Use memorable examples, illustrations, and elaborations.

4. Link your key points. Use minisummaries to repeat your major points. Gauge the audience's understanding with questions directed to them.

5. Begin preparations early. It always takes longer than anticipated to cover the literature, create interesting slides, and rehearse the presentation.

6. Consider including a patient case or a live patient as a jumping-off point for the discussion, whether you are giving a clinical or a research presentation. Attendees gain more when a patient case is woven into the presentation or a patient is present to answer questions about his or her presentation or illness. However, if a patient is coming to your presentation, take off at least ten minutes of your slide time to do the interview properly. Be sure to rehearse with the patient exactly what questions you will ask. Listen to the patient's answers over the phone or in person ahead of time to minimize surprises.

7. Make your presentation interactive by asking questions, using an audience-response system, scratch card answers, or "buzz groups" during the presentation (Cantillon 2003).

8. Conclude your presentation by covering the objectives and the key points attached to each.

9. Select, assort, and remove slides until your lecture slides and your

running commentary on them will easily fit the time allotted. Attendees will appreciate your starting and ending on time.

10. Provide a well-oiled, enthusiastic, clear distillation of your topic.

11. As a grand rounds presenter, you are the major "show person" of the week; prepare like a show person to engage the audience and teach excellent medicine.

12. Answer all questions with enthusiasm, poise, and patience, telling each person that the question is excellent, important, and pertinent, on the mark, cogent, or penetrating. Never become defensive, arrogant, or unpleasant. If a disagreement occurs, ask for the questioner's phone number or e-mail address so that you can send him or her the data you referred to, or say that you will look up the answer to the question. Smile and say thank you to the audience for being attentive and for participating in the learning experience.

Small-Group Learning Sessions at the Postgraduate Peer Level

Case-based learning is ideal for small groups of physicians, residents, and fellows (ten to thirty people) to have a wide-ranging discussion about an interesting clinical or research topic. Case-based learning, which business and law schools frequently use, is similar to problem-based learning except that in case-based learning the discussion is moved along by the discussion leaders' use of questions aimed at covering each of the case objectives (Garvin 2003).

The Mechanics

Elements of a small-group session are:

1. Make introductions.
2. Hand out the first page of the case.
3. Participants read aloud the case one page at a time. Be sure that you or your assistant collated the pages, one page at a time, in a stack separated by colorful blank pages, for easy distribution.
4. With your guidance, the group identifies facts, clarifies definitions and terms, and generates hypotheses and a learning agenda. You may wish to act as a scribe for the group, using a large standing flip chart and markers. This frees up the group for discussion.
5. Discuss the twists and turns of the case. Note the important points

of the history, physical examination, laboratory data, and x-rays that the group picks out.

6. The small-group learning at postgraduate meetings generally takes place in a conference room, with participants sitting at one, two, or three tables. As the discussion leader, you sit at the front table, if there is more than one table, and direct questions to all participants. Stand up if you need to answer a question directly or clarify a statement. Everyone in the room wants to hear your comments.

7. Be a catalyst and guide for a great discussion (Christensen 1991a, 1991b). Have your questions written out so that you can readily guide the participants toward a fruitful diagnosis, the multiple management options, the outcome of therapy, and conclusions (Kasulis 1984). Ideally, you will be able to elicit comments and opinions from each engaged participant in the room.

8. Hand out each case page after sufficient discussion has occurred.

9. End the session with a strong, clear summary of the participants' discussion and a schematic or slide set to solidify the important points; show evidence-based recommendations and take-home points (Greenwald 1991).

10. The leader brings each participant into the discussion if he or she has not entered within the first twenty minutes of a seventy-five- to ninety-minute case-based discussion.

Troubleshooting

If the goal of the small-group learning session is to learn as much as possible about the topic content, then it is preferable to hand out the objectives and initial pages of the case before the session to maximize preparation and participation. If the goal of the session is to see a group's ability to dissect a mystery case and come up with the answers using teamwork and group knowledge, without prior preparation, then the pages may be handed out as the case unfolds during the session. Traditionally, participants read the case aloud, one page at a time, so that each participant has the facts fresh in mind as the cooperative learning begins. The discussion leader has all visual aids ready. Although it is beneficial to the smooth running of the tutorial to have a predetermined series of questions to bring out important concepts during the discussion, the leader may not use many or all of these questions but may instead use others that come to mind to amplify and guide the discussion.

Questions may be used to move the discussion from one topic to another or to complete the discussion of important points. The discussion leader should prepare a short summary based on the stated objectives for the session. Design a helpful schematic or slide set to illustrate the concepts in the manner of a road map. The discussion leader may decide to summarize the discussion at certain points during the session, but he or she should leave enough time for a final summary.

Prepare intensively so that your session runs smoothly. Small groups foster the growth of communication skills and teamwork skills. You, as the leader, are responsible for making sure that no one person dominates and that every participant has a chance to speak. Effective small-group learning leads to vibrant and memorable discussions about real-life medical and scientific problems. These active-learning discussions solidify knowledge and improve understanding of key complex concepts.

✄ TEACHING TIPS

1. Write an interesting case, preferably based on a real patient case, with objectives, critical literature review, and excellent visual aids.
2. Create a set of slides to summarize important points and objectives to be covered in the discussion. The slide set will also include the visuals that accompany the case.
3. Create a handout of both the slide set and your literature review, with references.
4. Make sure that the room is not too small for the number of participants.
5. Manage small-group dynamics for the two major difficulties: the quiet learner and the dominant learner (Tiberius 1990). Ask questions of the quiet learner to bring him or her into the discussion. Turn your back to the dominant learner or overlook his or her raised hand to decrease the airtime for this person, and encourage others to take the floor by fixing your gaze on them.
6. Be sure to stop the discussion with enough time left to summarize. Give a slide summarizing discussion points at the end of the discussion. Let the group know from the beginning that you will give out the summary of the objectives at the end, including a handout with references. Saying this relaxes your participants. They can engage in conversation and not worry about taking notes.

Workshop Presentation

Participants expect to learn by doing in a workshop. Cochrane reviews of randomized controlled trials of educational methods indicate that the most effective educational methods are the most interactive (Satterlee, Eggers, and Grimes 2008). Set up your workshop to permit the participants to do two things: learn and work. Your workshop will be successful if you follow this advice. I know because the first workshop I gave was significantly marred by being a passive lecture, which provided little opportunity for participants to practice the techniques I was describing. Reviews were not good. I learned the hard way, and I went on to give well-received workshops after that painful experience.

Preparation for a workshop is critical.

1. The hardest part of a workshop preparation is to determine the action items.
2. Determine how long each action item will take so that you stay within the allotted time frame.
3. Create your handout materials using color and graphics to make them visually appealing and memorable (fig. 9.1).
4. Have nametags or cardboard nameplates at each participant's place to foster communication.
5. Present your didactic or explanatory background by minilecture or slide presentation within a fifteen-minute time slot in a ninety-minute session. Set aside the rest of the time for participants to explore and practice what you have just shown them.
6. Alert each participant and the group to the directions and the time limitations for the breakout work groups or individual exercises. Ask them to begin working. Tell them that you will be circulating among them to answer any questions.
7. Walk around to the tables, chairs, and seats of the participants looking over participants' shoulders and listening to what is going on. Volunteer to answer any questions.
8. At the end of the allotted time, ask each participant to explain his or her work, ideas, opinions, and work sheets to the group (fig. 9.1). This feedback, which frequently takes more time than allotted, is the participants' favorite and the most memorable part of the workshop, as they listen to interesting new ideas and solutions given by their col-

	Create a story line around one of these symptoms and signs (or make up one of your own):
Becoming Aware	1. Exertional chest pain 4. Headaches
	2. Wheezing 5. Chronic renal failure
	3. Rectal bleeding 6. Fatigue
	7. Other
Health care disparities have been noted amongst a wide range of patient populations: African-Americans Asian-Americans Hispanic-Americans Native-Americans/ Pacific Islanders Women Poor Disabled Non-English Speaking Elderly Illiterate Gays/Lesbians Obese Religious Groups Alcohol and Substance Abusers Illegal Immigrants Alternative medicine users **Factors to consider:** Stereotyping Cultural contrasts Racial disparities Socioeconomic biases Health care outcomes Alternative lifestyles Dietary diversity Complementary medicine Language barriers and need for interpreters	Add "triggers" to the story line to promote discussion of racial/cultural/ethnic/socioeconomic issues. List questions to promote discussion of your "triggers."

Figure 9.1. **Worksheet for Becoming Aware of Cultural Differences and Similarities and Creating Cases for Educational Use**

Use the worksheet to help create scenarios with embedded triggers that will stimulate the discussion of cultural, racial, ethnic, and socioeconomic factors in preclinical or clinical small groups, laboratories, or tutorials.

Source: Produced by Helen Shields, Jane Hayward, and Vinod Nambudiri, 2008.

leagues. This is what participants have signed up for: new knowledge, ideas, and enthusiasm.

9. If time is running short, do not drop an action item, just explain that, although time is short, you value their trying the exercise even if they do not get all the way through it. This gives participants a sense of your commitment to their education and your enthusiasm. You are respecting their time.

10. Remember that participants have paid money to come to your workshop. Make it worthwhile. Have an excellent bibliography and a slide-set handout and worksheet handouts that look professionally done.

11. Obtain immediate and final feedback so that you can solidify what you did well and correct what went wrong.

12. Workshop participants should be all smiles if you have taught them a new method or approach to an educational problem and they have had the opportunity to try to make it work for them.

13. Give your business card to each participant. Say you will stay after the session to speak with anyone who has a question or comment.

Directing a Postgraduate Course

The position of postgraduate course director is an honor and an opportunity to appear on national or international teaching stages. However, it also has the potential to be an educational disaster because all eyes will eventually be on the course evaluations that are made known to the sponsoring organization, the governing board, and a host of other people. You are competing with all course directors who have gone before you and all who will come after you. You are generally chosen eighteen months ahead of time, so you can observe the course before yours and develop a unique and competitive program that reflects the needs assessment your organization has made concerning topics of interest to members. Your work will be extensive over the eighteen months, rising steadily to a crescendo at the time the course you are directing begins. You will learn many good and important teaching lessons, but you will also spend a great deal of time working without much pay (except for a modest standard honorarium). Having been a co–course director for a large postgraduate course will be another educational notch on your CV, but it may not be worth the great investment of time. Make sure you have extraordinarily effective administrators and co–course directors to help make the numerous planning decisions less onerous.

✄ TEACHING TIPS

1. The success of this position is directly linked to the course administrator. Weak administration will not be offset by your strengths as a clinician, educator, or researcher.

2. The course director decides on the course curriculum in concert with the governing board of the organization sponsoring the course. Once the topics have been agreed on, choose lecturers and small-group leaders with the utmost care. Review past evaluations and personal recollections of lectures given by the nominated faculty to help make decisions.

3. Issue invitations by a personal phone call to potential speakers. If a speaker cannot lecture at that time and place, ask him or her to suggest a substitute. The substitute may or may not have the same cachet as the original invited speaker.

4. Once a speaker accepts, he or she is sent a contract and notification of the honorarium as well as the slide set and handout requirements.

5. Speakers will occasionally pull out close to the time of the course owing to personal or health reasons. This puts a pressing burden on the course directors to quickly find another excellent speaker.

6. The course director oversees the review of all materials and slide sets before they go to the publisher.

7. Carefully scrutinize conflicts of interest and industry ties with respect to the lecture and slide material. If bias is found, ask the speaker to revise the presentation and send it back for rereview to check that the slides or handout materials are well balanced and without a conflict of interest.

8. Course directors need to select room sizes in convention halls based on estimates of attendees.

9. Course directors should plan on being at the entire course to troubleshoot all problems that arise.

10. Give direct instructions to each speaker about the allotted time for presentation, about objectives, and about slide set requirements. Review all slides for content, conflict of interest, and correct referencing of data. Note the number of slides because frequently too many slides are being submitted to fit the allotted time. Ask the presenter to delete some slides. Volunteer to help him or her make the final choice.

11. Give presentation tips and frequently reiterate the need to stay within the allotted time slot.

12. Learn the biographical information that you will use in your introduction of the speaker at the podium. Put this streamlined factual information on a 3 x 5 inch card. Do not hesitate to read it from the card or memorize it rather than be inaccurate.

13. On site, familiarize yourself with the podium, the media specialists up front, and the microphone system, light system, and type of screen that will show the slides and the teleprompter, if there is one.

14. Delegate what you know others can do well; otherwise, guard your reputation as an organized and effective educator and administrator by trying to stay on top of problems as they arise.

15. Be pleasant, no matter how many problems arise; continue to think of creative solutions until the last talk has been given.

16. Smile and look confident even if things are going wrong; those around you will mirror your mood. They need to continue to work hard despite the glitches that have occurred.

17. Avoid backbiting and blaming when the ratings come out. Give it your all while the process is going on. No regrets is best.

18. Make a plan for the course director group following you, if the position rotates yearly. If you have the option of repeating as course director, devise a solution to each of the difficulties identified in the course evaluations and ask for personnel to help you make the necessary changes.

19. Be appreciative and pleasant concerning of all your speakers' efforts, even if a speaker falls short of your expectations. You will continue to see these people for the rest of your career.

20. Thank the person who appointed you to the course-director position in writing before the evaluations are known. You are grateful for the opportunity and the experience, even if the evaluations are less than stellar and he or she is disappointed at not topping the best prior ratings for this annual course.

Moderating a Clinical or Research Forum at a National Meeting

The moderator is expected to introduce the program and guide the discussion. In addition, as a moderator, you may be responsible for choosing the program for the forum by reading all the abstracts and grading their worthiness to be either a poster or an oral presentation. You help choose the final "best" abstracts for oral presentation, and you will sit on the dais or platform during the presentation of this abstract session, introducing each speaker and the title of the presentation, fielding and asking questions, and keeping time. You may be called on to give short introductions of topics and presenters. You are also expected to clearly articulate the goals of the session, lead the discussion, and encourage audience participation (Sisco 1998). Take your duties seriously because it means so much to the abstract presenter to have a knowledgeable and respectful moderator. Practice reading out loud the names of the presenters the day or evening before the session you are moderating. If you are uncertain about a pronunciation, ask the presenter, before he or she comes to the podium, how to pronounce the name. Remember to read all the abstracts that pertain to the area of interest of your session. Conflicting data may be being presented. You need to be aware of these conflicts so that you can lead an excellent discussion of the opposing points of view.

TEACHING TIPS

1. Research the topics in your session to decide who should be accepted for presentation or for poster. Become even more of an expert in the field.

2. Once the program is settled, read the literature on the accepted abstracts for which you will be moderating the discussion.

3. Dress well for the moderator role. You will likely have a picture taken of you on the stage.

4. Practice the pronunciation of the presenters' names, title of the presentation, and the sponsoring university or organization out loud the evening before. If you are uncertain of a pronunciation, find the presenter in the audience before the session begins and ask how to pronounce the name, title, or university or organization.

5. Write out, on a 3 x 5 or 5 x 7 inch index card, questions for each of the accepted oral presentation abstracts. Keep these cards with you. Review the questions and consider changing them after you have seen new data that may emerge at the meeting from other laboratories or groups.

6. Arrive thirty minutes early to the room, even if another session is ongoing, to see its size. Look for steps to the podium that are uneven or steep and alert speakers to any danger before they try to mount the steps in a semi-darkened room.

7. Introduce yourself to the media specialist; ask where lights, microphone, and pointer are.

8. Keep time; practice using the official timer; help presenters with microphone and lights.
9. Always smile and be pleasant to presenters; you are not presenting—they are—and they need your friendly support as moderator.
10. If a questioner from the audience becomes rude or aggressive, cut him or her off and go to the next questioner or ask a prepared question.
11. Shake hands with your co-moderator, if you have one, at the beginning and at the end of the session. Tell him or her how much you enjoyed sharing the podium.
12. Make mental notes for what you would do differently the next time.

Poster Presentations

Poster presenters are frequently disappointed by not being assigned the more glamorous oral presentation. However, if a poster presenter takes the opportunity seriously to present his or her data over a ten-hour period, he or she will find interesting and profitable interactions with peers, future mentors, and competitors. The following suggestions will help you maximize your educational learning from a poster presentation.

✂ TEACHING TIPS

1. If the poster session opens at 8 a.m. in the hall or convention center, set up your poster promptly at 8 a.m., or earlier, so that you can catch attendees as they go into the poster area before attending the meetings.
2. Because it will be a long day of intermittent standing, wear comfortable shoes and be sure to eat breakfast and lunch.
3. Have a notebook to take down attendees' questions, suggestions, and criticisms.
4. Prepare a summary of your poster and memorize it. Consider preparing a long, complete summary and a shorter abbreviated version of your data.
5. After introducing yourself to each person who stops at your poster, ask whether he or she prefers the long or short version of your summary.
6. Walk the person through your poster data, focusing on its highlights and importance to your field.
7. If the person does not want a summary of your data, but prefers to look at it for him- or herself, say that you would be happy to answer any questions about the data or methodology.

8. Have prepared answers to expected questions and possible methodological or study design issues.

9. If there are other posters on similar topics, discuss how your poster fits in.

10. Write down any possible future collaboration with attendees. Ask for e-mail addresses or business cards and put them in your notebook. Make business cards of your own with your e-mail address and location to hand out to prospective collaborators.

11. Do not be afraid to question attendees as to whether they are working in the same field. These competitor attendees may be a fountain of information.

12. Always be pleasant, even if negative comments are made about your data.

13. Remember that you are the salesperson of your data and its message. Enjoy selling your interesting results.

14. View the poster session as one continuous question-and-answer period, in which you will educate others and learn from your audience.

15. Recognize that the poster session is an opportunity to identify and network with potential collaborators from other institutions and hospitals.

Ten-Minute Platform Presentations

You have just received the e-mail message that your abstract for a national meeting has been chosen for a ten-minute platform presentation. You feel great; this is a definite high point marked by pride and excitement, particularly when you are a junior faculty member, fellow, or resident. The tremendous excitement and pride rapidly gives way, however, to abject terror as you picture yourself on the podium of the national meeting. You imagine yourself flubbing a question asked by a competitor. You see the disappointment on your mentor's face as your mind goes blank when you are asked about the specifics of the methodology. You feel the cold palms and red face as your slide set will not project, or another speaker's slide set is loaded in your slot and you have no idea where your slide set is. All of these awful scenarios are possible and do occur; that is why you and your mentor or your colleagues, research group, and family and friends will spend a great deal of time preparing you for your platform presentation. If you are a mid-level or senior faculty member, you should seek the help of a trustworthy and honest person familiar with the field and ask him or her to listen to your presentation and explanations to hypothetical questions.

Rehearsal Is Essential

Focused preparation and hours of practice are the keys to a relatively worry-free presentation. I say "relatively" because no one is without some fear concerning a platform presentation, largely because of the element of uncertainty about the level and depth of the questions that could be asked during the five minutes following a classic ten-minute presentation. Although the same questions could be asked of the poster presenter, the public forum, the larger audience, the microphone, and the possibility of taping add to the concern about the swiftness, accuracy, and confidence of your answers. On the other hand, extensive and intensive preparations should completely eliminate all worries regarding the presentation slides, staying within the allotted time frame, knowing your methods backward and forward, as well as the data set and analyses and the current literature. After all, you have practiced in front of your research group, your department, and your mentor. You have timed yourself and been timed. Many criticisms later, your slide set is as clear as it can be, and you have memorized certain phrases concerning your methodology and why you chose it. How do you get to the stage where you feel that the only variable is uncertainty about the particular questions that will be asked? You should have no uncertainty about expected questions, because your friends, colleagues, and mentors should have been peppering you with easy, medium, and hard questions from the beginning. Easy questions may be related to technique; medium questions relate to why you chose the particular model you did or the appropriateness of the control group, while harder questions focus on your speculation concerning the work's significance or why the data you are presenting are diametrically opposed to another group's data.

The following tips will help you give a memorable and trouble-free presentation at a major meeting. You want to feel proud, elated, and ready to pat yourself on the back, rather than feeling deflated and guilt-ridden at the end of your platform presentation. You wish to walk off the podium with your head held high rather than slink back to your seat after botching the answers to several key questions from rival groups.

✂ TEACHING TIPS

1. **As soon as you receive the notice of your acceptance for the platform presentation, alert your mentor, your group, and your family. Although the presentation is generally two to three months away, you have a new**

and important deadline to focus on, one that requires adjusting your calendar to make space for rehearsals, revisions, and memorization.

2. Set up a schedule for rehearsals with your mentor, your research colleagues, or your laboratory partners. At initial rehearsals, focus on the data to show, the photographs to display, and the summary and conclusions to announce to the research community. At subsequent rehearsals have a group of colleagues critique each of your tentative slides for their utility, accuracy, simplicity, and visual impact across a large room.

3. Review the other topics and data being presented in your session and in related platform sessions or poster sessions so that obvious discrepancies in data and conclusions can be discussed ahead of time. You will likely be asked about differences between what you and other groups are presenting. Be ready to explain what may have led to the differences.

4. Watch your time limits. If you have ten minutes, you should have no more than eight to ten slides, including the title and acknowledgment slides. Trying to explain fifteen to eighteen slides in a ten-minute time slot will only confuse and annoy your audience.

5. Prepare intensively for the early rehearsals by writing out each word that you will say, including your introductory comments to the moderators of the session, who announce your name, the names of your co-investigators, and the title of your abstract. The simplest and best initial comment may be "Thank you, Dr. Smith and Dr. Jones" or "Dr. Smith, Dr. Jones, members, and guests." Generally, you can find the names of the moderators of your session a few weeks before the meeting in the tentative program. Otherwise, the program book that you are given when you arrive usually has the moderators' names in it. Use these names and learn how to pronounce them from colleagues who are familiar with the moderators.

6. Write out a separate sheet, in a large font, for each slide so that, if you have not memorized it or are worried about forgetting it in the heat of battle, you can turn each slide page over on the podium the day of the talk.

7. Launch into your first slide, which is your disclosure slide, noting "I have no disclosures to make" or "I have no conflicts of interest" or "I have been supported by X, Y, and Z."

8. Begin your presentation with a background slide asking the question you posed for yourself when you began the project to let the audience know why you performed your project. The background slide sets the stage for your hypothesis.

9. Outline your aims simply and clearly, using bullets or numbers to organize the aims in the order of both priority and logic of research plan.

10. State the methods.

11. Show the results in table or figure form. Use color to distinguish important points. Avoid complexity in the results section.

12. Do not strive to be complete in the demonstration of your data sets. Rather, carefully pick and choose your data to make the most effective talk for a discussion. This is an expository talk, not an in-depth publication.

13. Walk the audience through your results, explaining your group's thinking about the data and its implications.

14. State the summary of the project.

15. List one, two, or three conclusions, if these are different from your summary.

16. Show an acknowledgment slide for all your co-workers, mentors, and grant or foundation support.

17. Thank the audience at the end to indicate you have concluded your presentation, then wait for the applause.

18. Have pencil and paper at the podium to jot down questions you are being asked, particularly multipart questions. Repeat the question as part of your answer. Members of the audience who did not hear or understand the question are then able to appreciate your answer and follow the discussion.

19. The day of or the day before, check the room size and placement of the podium and familiarize yourself with the media specialist or audiovisual person who will help you. Check that your slide set is where it should be. If not, ask for immediate help.

20. Practice using the laser pointer for slides that require you to point out a significant finding. If your hand shakes, consider having an arrow put on the slide; you will not have to point but you will need to memorize a phrase, for example, "The arrow in the right corner shows the important change that occurred."

21. Get your sleep the night before. Eat ahead of time, but avoid gassy

foods and carbonated sodas, which may lead to burping and bloating at inopportune times.

22. Wear your best outfit for a business occasion. Make sure it is also flattering to you.
23. Wear comfortable shoes. Beware of high heels getting stuck in a platform makeshift staircase.

✒ TAKE-HOME POINTS

- Postgraduate audiences expect value for their time and money; give it to them.
- Send a copy of your talk by e-mail or CD to the person sponsoring your lecture to see if the talk will open and can be projected; you will never regret taking the time to do this.
- Practice your lecture out loud; ask nonmedical friends to listen for delivery, clarity, and logical flow.
- Select, sort, and delete slides until your presentation comfortably fits the time slot. Never apologize for a crowded slide; don't show it.
- Never put anything on a slide or say anything that could be offensive to anyone.
- Summarize your main objectives at the end of your lecture.
- Case-based learning requires an active discussion leader; become this leader, who questions, listens, and responds.
- Workshop participants want to be active as part of the learning; create action items that are fun and educational.
- Being a course director for a large postgraduate course is an honor, but it is also time-consuming; before accepting the position, make sure the administrators working with you are capable and industrious.
- Scrutinize all presentations, as the course director, for potential conflict-of-interest problems; ask some speakers to revise their slides and handouts after you have carefully reviewed them.
- As a moderator at a national meeting, research the topics in your session; write questions on index cards so that you can ask a question if not enough questions come from the audience.
- Enjoy your poster presentation as one long question-and-answer period in which you have the luxury of interacting with potential collaborators.
- Rehearse for a platform presentation to enjoy your victory on the stage.

CHAPTER TEN

Additional Teaching Methods

- ✂ *What is team-based learning?*
- ✂ *Are there objective data to show that this method works to improve learning and learner satisfaction?*
- ✂ *What is cross-cultural care, and how do I integrate it into learning exercises?*
- ✂ *Are simulation exercises of value to trainees?*
- ✂ *What is a multistation exercise, and when is it most effective?*
- ✂ *How do I give an excellent journal club presentation?*
- ✂ *What are objective structured teaching exercises?*

Definition of Team-based Learning

We recently introduced team-based learning into the laboratories of the gastrointestinal pathophysiology course as a method for increasing the interest and engagement in these important teaching exercises, which do not have required attendance. Students were enthusiastic, and voluntary attendance was high. Eighty to ninety percent of the expected students were at each of the three laboratories. The student rumor mill placed these labs as "high yield" in the students' preboard studying parlance. Student and faculty feedback was excellent.

I had observed two of Dr. Daniel Mayer's classes at Albany Medical College to learn the methodology. Dr. Mayer's name was listed on the Team-Based Learning Collaborative Web site (www.tblcollaborative.org) as a resource for those who sought to learn how to incorporate team-based learning into preclinical courses. I came away from my one-day visit with firsthand knowledge of a new medical education technique, which subsequently worked well in our pathology laboratories, engaging forty students from the moment they walked into one of the four large classrooms until the end of the 90- to 110-minute sessions.

Team-based learning is an example of active learning that allows a single teacher to teach multiple small groups simultaneously in the same classroom (Allen and Tanner 2005). Team-based learning is an excellent way to teach a large group, using a method that combines small-group interactive learning with an expert teacher giving desired content (Michaelsen and Sweet 2008a, 2008b; Parmelee 2008; Parmelee, DeStephen, and Borges 2009). It has been touted as a useful new learning tool that involves teams in small-group learning experiences within a large classroom setting.

The method involves dividing a class into independent small groups (Haidet, O'Malley, and Richards 2002). Each group learns identical assigned objectives, using materials provided by the instructor. At the beginning of class, learners are given a test called the Individual Readiness Assurance Test (IRAT), which gives the instructor an idea of each student's preparation. Later in the class, the same or a similar test, called the Group Readiness Assurance Test (GRAT), is given to the group for a consensus response. The groups' answers are developed after individual group discussion. Classroom technology is available for "on-the-spot feedback." Methods for quickly documenting the responses of groups include the use of color-coded cards, scratch tickets, clickers, and wireless hand-held response pads. The answers can be captured, stored, and graphed quickly for sharing with the student groups. Once the groups' answers have been decided on, the correct answers are provided. Following this, all the groups exchange information and try to jointly solve the problems posed. Team-based learning encourages addressing the learning objectives and evaluating the level of knowledge of the learners and permits the instructor to correct misconceptions. Students can compare the success of their group with that of others, and they do group problem solving. It is essential that students prepare outside class and bring their knowledge and theories to the group process. Class time is slanted toward application and integration of information. The instructor acts as a content expert and facilitator. Both individual and team performances are recognized. The method promotes accountability.

Team-based learning is similar to problem-based learning in that a small group works with a facilitator to learn content. It differs because the instructor is the expert for multiple groups rather than just one group. The problem-based learning student-to-teacher ratio is usually about eight students to one teacher, while in team-based learning the ratio may be as high as two hundred students to one teacher. Team-based learning also differs by using the initial readiness assurance test to emphasize prior preparation. Students in problem-based learning groups are encouraged to prepare beforehand to enrich the discussion, but the team-based approach makes the stakes higher for prior preparation by having quizzes that count for both the individual and for the group at the beginning of each session. In addition, groups complete assignments in class and simultaneously compare their answers, thus receiving immediate feedback. In problem-based learning, students make a learning agenda during each session that is to be completed outside class. At the end of team-based learning, there is another test, a group assurance readiness test. In problem-based learning, there is no check during the session to make sure that each student has grasped the basic concepts, whereas this is a central tenet for the team-based learning. Problem-based learning groups are typically led by a student but encouraged by the facilitator, who may or may not be a content expert, to stay on track, cover the unfolding story, and make decisions about the material presented. In contrast, in team-based learning, one teacher, who is a content expert, moves medium and large groups of students through complex problems and solutions.

Team-based learning has been shown to lead to increased student engagement (Kelly et al. 2005) and to foster student participation and group assessment. This method can be applied to any scientific discipline, from pharmacology to cell biology or pathology. It has been touted as useful in helping students acquire skills in the interpretation of experimental data, in answering probing questions, and in assessing themselves for understanding content, thus showing accountability for their studying.

The initial investment of time is considerable. Time is spent creating materials and making up assessment questions for the initial assessment and summary group assessment. However, a similar amount of time may be spent on creating a problem-based learning case. Once the team-based learning exercise has been created, it may be used over and over again, with variations similar to the problem-based learning case.

The benefits of shifting to team-based learning from the usual lecture format are multiple. Team-based learning has been shown to improve communication and problem solving and to increase student engagement compared to a lecture course. Students feel that it increases their preclass participation and gives improved insight into the materials. They appreciate the teamwork skills and respect for colleagues who have different viewpoints. Team-based learning creates a positive attitude toward out-of-class preparation and increases student accountability. The risks of this teaching model are that students may worry about directing their own learning and feel that, although they are engaged, they may not be learning as much content.

Although several medical education researchers have looked for objective evidence of a better learning outcome with team-based learning, they have not found it. National test scores have not improved. Student attitudes toward learning may be better, but objective scores are not. Parmelee et al.'s (2009) article supports this, showing that first- and second-year medical students (N = 180) do not report a significant benefit for team-based education in helping them learn course material better. These students, however, did agree with being satisfied overall with the team experience in year one (4.13) and year two (4.24) on a Likert Scale of 1–5, in which 5 is "agree strongly" and 4 is "agree." They rated the team experience as significantly improving from year one to year two (p = 0.024). Of interest, and as yet unexplained, is Parmelee et al.'s (2009) data indicating from year one to year two that satisfaction with peer evaluation went down, as did the students' perceived usefulness of working in a team to develop skills in professional development (p <. 001).

Team-based learning has had many modifications and has been used in many different professional school and hospital settings since its introduction, by Larry Michaelsen, in the 1970s (Al-Mateen 2008; Dunaway 2005; Kitchen et al. 2003). I watched an online video of one of Dr. Michaelsen's classes through the team-based learning collaborative Web site (www.tblcollaborative.org) and found it exciting and challenging to see one teacher conduct an engaging learning experience for so many students. The essential elements of team-based learning are thoughtful group formation and nurturing of the groups, student accountability for their own and group work, regular feedback, and assignments that encourage learning of content and foster group development. The instructor should construct groups so that each is primed for success by the diverse skills of its members. Groups remain the same for the entire course of instruction, so each team member can exhibit his or her particular skills over time. Avoid cliques forming within groups because they are disruptive to group function. Readiness assurance tests promote preparation by the individual student and contribute to the quality of the discussion by the group. Assignments for the group should encourage group decision-making rather than be solvable by the individual student.

Dr. Michaelsen spends a significant amount of time and energy making up the teams for his classes (Michaelsen and Sweet 2008a, 2008b), which are composed of five to seven people and which take advantage of different student backgrounds and strengths, gender, ethnicity, communication style, and socialization (2008). Linked and mutually reinforcing assignments are essential to success. Dr. Michaelsen notes that the maximum "learning payoff" occurs when the 3 S's are followed (although many subsequent copies of the method do not use the 3 S's) (2008). The 3 S's are:

1. Same problem: Groups work on the same problem.
2. Specific choice: Groups are required to use course materials to make a specific choice.
3. Simultaneously report: Whenever possible, groups report their choices simultaneously by holding up cards denoting the correct answer.

A large classroom is sufficient for team-based learning. Ideally, chairs should be movable, to create different areas for groupings to occur. Visibility is a key strategy, so answers held up on large cards must be able to be readily seen.

Integration of Cross-cultural Care into Teaching a Preclinical Course

Cross-cultural or culturally competent care refers to understanding how cultural and social differences affect patients and their experience of illness. Disparities in health care on the basis of race, socioeconomic status, and ethnicity are well recognized. Promoting cross-cultural care early and often in the preclinical years is one way to try to have students and faculty members gain the knowledge, skills, and attitudes necessary for them to care for the diverse populations they will serve (Betancourt 2003; Sequist 2009). In addition, through education, students and faculty may recognize their own biases (Kumagai and Lypson 2009). One hopes that this recognition will eventually decrease disparities. The discussions of cultural and social issues should focus on their relevance to health care. Ho and colleagues (2008) showed that inpatient-centered cultural competency training could produce improvement in medical students' cross-cultural communication skills as measured by an objective structured clinical examination (OSCE).

Bringing cross-cultural care into preclinical teaching sessions, lectures, or large- or small-group case-discussion sessions requires a strong commitment to finding relevant and compelling inter-relationships between cultural and ethnic material and the medical science you and your faculty are trying to teach. Medical students were the first to urge me to bring cultural and ethnic issues into the gastrointestinal pathophysiology course (Saha et al. 2008). I resisted because I did not understand what the words meant, or their significance. Later, I researched the literature and began to understand the magnitude of health care disparities and the possible benefit of introducing medical students to a discussion of cultural, racial, and socioeconomic factors during tutorial. It took us several years to devise a faculty development program that had enough buy-in from the tutors to make a significant difference in the tutors' active discussion of cross-cultural care topics in the tutorial (Shields and Leffler et al. 2009). Many of the faculty, like me, initially thought that trying to teach pathophysiology and discuss ethnic, cultural, and socioeconomic factors would be difficult. The key was to find cultural factors that were relevant to the science we, as tutors, were trying to convey. While the students were ready, willing, and able to discuss both topics, the tutors had more difficulty (Shields and Nambudiri et al. 2009). This is why it is important to direct your initial efforts at faculty and choose relevant cultural factors for the pathophysiology under discussion. Cultural factors need to have a central importance in the case if discussions about them are to take place.

The Mechanics of Developing a Cross-cultural Care Initiative for Preclinical Teaching

1. Develop new case material or alter existing case material to add "triggers." Triggers are social, racial, ethnic, or socioeconomic factors that are relevant to the scientific aims of the cases. Some examples of triggers that we used are the surreptitious use of alternative medicine (Wetzel, Kaptchuk, and Eisenberg 2003), inability to pay for essential medication, obesity, alcoholism, and ethnic and cultural foods that are detrimental to a patient's health. Deciding on which triggers to use and how to develop discussion of both science and culture requires a great deal of thought and discussion on the part of the teachers who are developing these curricular materials.

2. Assessment of cross-cultural care triggers by a student group or a committee may be helpful. At Harvard Medical School, the student subcommittee of the Cross-Cultural Care Committee reviewed each of our three tutorial cases for the cultural aspects of the case and provided us with pertinent and valuable insights into what would work and what would not (Shields and Nambudiri et al. 2009). The students' suggestions were almost uniformly used. Each student was acknowledged on the copyrighted case. Tutors and students were more likely to actively discuss the triggers once they knew that a stu-

dent group had vetted the triggers in the cases and agreed with their importance and relevance.

3. Faculty development is key to ensuring the success of this important teaching exercise because the faculty is already worried about teaching the science and you are requesting that they also teach about cultural and ethnic issues (Shields and Leffler et al. 2009).

Specific Faculty Development Program for the Integration of Cross-cultural Care

Use a one-hour faculty development session to get your faculty to understand your goals and their importance. I recommend a brisk, fast-paced, five-part session to hold the attention of your faculty and encourage them to take ownership of this material (Shields and Leffler et al. 2009). Multiple teachers and experts may be involved in teaching the one-hour session, or the head of the course can do it all.

A few days before the faculty development session, hand out the case material with the trigger elements bolded in an e-mail attachment or by hard copy, giving the faculty time to preview it.

The components of a faculty development session are:

1. Begin the session with a five-minute overview of the importance of cross-cultural care by a knowledgeable expert or experts.
2. Move on to a discussion by the course director on disparities in health care, with slides showing pertinent references that are relevant to the organ system and diseases that are being taught.
3. Divide the teachers into several small groups to discuss the bolded cases and to develop questions to use in their own tutorial groups to promote the discussion of the case triggers. These questions will be shared with all tutors. Assign each group a different case, if possible, and ask that each group elect a person to speak for the group. At the end of a fifteen-minute interval, the questions generated by each group are put on the blackboard or overhead projector or computer and projected for all to see. These questions are copied for distribution to the tutors before the official tutorial sessions begin.
4. The course director or designated teacher should discuss the interweaving of the science, medicine, and cultural and ethnic issues with

the use of slides, blackboard, or overhead projector presentation of the trigger relevance for each case and how to frame its importance for the students. This should take ten minutes.

5. During the final twenty minutes of the session, faculty views a video made of a mock tutorial, with real students and a real tutor discussing the alcoholism trigger from the tutorial case of end-stage cirrhosis. Tutors are able to discuss and reflect on what occurs in the mock group and try to anticipate how they will be able to replicate the relaxed discussion by the students and the use of probing questions by the tutor.

6. Tutors are given references for each of the trigger elements and handouts to help them understand cross-cultural care and its importance.

Simulation-based Training

After the Institute of Medicine Report on medical errors, *To Err Is Human* (Kohn, Corrigan, and Donaldson 1999), physicians became more aware of the importance of performance-based assessment and the use of simulation-based training to achieve competency in certain areas (Issenberg et al. 1999; Issenberg et al. 2005). Miller's (1990) pyramid depicts the methods of learning and assessment of a graduating physician using the four increasing levels, from "knowledge" to "knows how" to "shows how" to "does," independently at the top of the pyramid. McGaghie (1999) defined simulation as a person, device, or set of conditions that attempts to present education and evaluation problems authentically. Often the student or trainee responds to problems as he or she would under normal circumstances and receives feedback on the performance. Simulation models are one way of training and then assessing performance so that the graduate or trainee will achieve Miller's "does" independently at a high level. Scott et al. (2008) showed a certification rate of 100 percent for laparoscopic surgery skills after two months of simulation training. None of the trainees passed the certification test before the simulation training. Other studies have shown benefit from these simulation-based training exercises, including mastering skills that are directly transferable to real patient situations (Barsuk et al. 2009; Wayne et al. 2005). A study of simulation-based mastery of placement of central venous catheters showed that the simulation-trained subjects had higher success and fewer complications than an observational control group (Barsuk et al. 2009). However, in an editorial accompanying this article, Appavu (2009) points out that the number of insertions performed by each of the study subjects in Barsuk's study was small. Another study by Wayne et al. (2005), which focused on a randomized trial of improving skills with a simulator for advanced life support, also showed that the simulator training improved skills compared to a group that did not receive this simulator training.

I have used simulation training during the gastrointestinal pathophysiology course to help second-year students gain a mastery of the classic approach to the diagnosis and management of an upper gastrointestinal bleeder and a lower gastrointestinal bleeder. Students work though each case at the bedside of a high-fidelity robot mannequin. Scripts must be created for the mannequin, consultants, and each of the nurses or doctors who will be involved in the case. In addition, laboratory data, x-rays, and endoscopic materials of high quality need to be interwoven into the case in a realistic manner. Students discuss the case among themselves and then present to the endoscopy fellow and "attending" their findings and their differential diagnoses and plans. Some students find the simulation exercises an excellent bridge to their clinical clerkships the following year. Others enjoy the ability to share out loud their budding differential diagnosis skills and praise the comfortable setting that permits them to gain confidence in thinking about medical problems.

Andreatta and Gruppen (2009) emphasized the importance of validity evidence in the assessment process for simulation-based medical training and have provided a logical framework to structure the type and degree of validity evidence. The jury is still out on the long-term retention of the simulation-based procedural skills. Appavu (2009) calls for better-designed prospective multicenter studies, encompassing larger numbers of subjects, and standardization of simulation equipment to try to demonstrate the benefits of simulation.

Integrated Multistation Exercises

Of all the teaching exercises I have been involved with over the years, the one that receives the most praise and brings the most smiles is the integrated multistation exercise. What is it and why is it so popular? Integrated multistation exercises were developed by Miriam S. Wetzel, PhD, and Lynne M. Reid, MD, at Harvard Medical School in the early 1990s (Wetzel and Reid 1991; Zimmerman, Ruben, and Ahwesh 2005; McArdle, 2007). The clinical scenarios encourage active small-group learning of clinically relevant material, with a limited amount of faculty time. This method can be used in both the preclinical and clinical years and is suited to curricula driven by objectives. The method consists of a series of physically separated stations in a laboratory or skills area where high-quality visual exhibits (including EKGs, x-rays, photomicrographs, and gross and microscopic pathology specimens, enlarged and mounted on posterboard-size sheets of thick paper) are taped on the laboratory walls or on cabinet doors. These large exhibits are coupled with history, physical examination, and laboratory data, which are also mounted and pasted on the laboratory cabinets for ease of viewing. The integrated multistation preclinical exercises encourage small groups of students to pull together major concepts in several organ systems simultaneously. They are particularly popular in the middle and at the end of a physiology or pathophysiology course and are usually held up as a prime method for integrating material from disparate organs, such as the esophagus, kidney, and musculoskeletal system. This type of preclinical exercise lasts for two to two and one-half hours, with approximately equal amounts of time spent discussing the cases in the individual groups and presenting them to the whole group, with both student and faculty commentary.

Before beginning this exercise, the class or resident group is broken into groups of equal size. Each group of about forty students or residents meets in a large classroom to receive instructions about number of stations (usually three to four), time limit (twenty to twenty-five minutes per station), and individual and group responsibilities. Then groups of students or residents are dispersed to the individual stations, which are duplicated in each skills area, so no more than five to ten people are working on a station at one time. A duplicate group is working on the same station in a different geographic area within the same skills area. Groups begin working their way clockwise around the three to four exhibit areas. One faculty member can interact with groups ranging from ten students to thirty residents. Expert consultants circulate among groups as the official timekeepers, listen to the learners' interactive discussions, and provide some direction, if needed. The faculty consultant is asked not to "give away" the case at this point in the exercise. The underlying aim of these exercises is to encourage teamwork and dialogue, leading to a better understanding of pathophysiologic concepts or complex clinical scenarios.

At the end of the allotted time, a "time is up" signal is called out, and the group of participants moves to the next station. A few more minutes are given to the last station so that each group can choose a presenter and prepare a summary of the case's pathophysiology. Once all stations have been viewed, participants move into a central classroom or auditorium to discuss each case and explain the concepts with the help of the teaching faculty. Each team brings the last case history, along with the readily movable exhibits, into the classroom and tapes them up on the blackboards and whiteboards around the room. One of the two teams that just finished viewing and discussing the exhibits and history and laboratory data is asked to nominate a designated presenter. This designated presenter gives a short summary of the team's collective explanation of the case from his or her seat or by standing in front of the exhibits and describing the group's thought processes as well as the underlying pathophysiologic concepts. Each group is also asked to jointly arrive at the case "solution" and make this known to the teaching faculty during the presentation.

As each presenter finishes, the rest of the large group is asked if anyone has questions, comments, or disagreements with what has been said. The faculty rates each group on the accuracy of the "solution" and overall quality of the presentation. The faculty may add explanations, ask questions of the group, or bring in connections that have been missed or misunderstood. Teaching faculty discuss each case after students from other teams ask questions or add explanations. The faculty's role is to make connections the students may have missed and answer any lingering questions the students may have before the final examination. Illumination rather than obfuscation should be the order of the day. Faculty give concise, clear explanations and are honored for their ability to make complex concepts understandable, especially because these integrated multistation exercises are often close to exam time in the preclinical years and are good preparation for specialty board exams in the clinical years.

Journal Club Presentations

A journal club presentation provides an opportunity to show off your critical evaluative skills, whether you are the presenter or the faculty consultant for a resident's journal club (Alguire 1998; Edwards, Woolf, and Hetzler 2002; Linzer et al. 1988). Is the original research article destined to be a classic? Does it suffer from poor methodology, inaccurate statistical analyses, or flawed data sets? I prefer to spend my precious time preparing and discussing a "great" article, though I have a number of colleagues who delight in finding "flawed" articles to take apart and delineate the research methodology problems. Decide which camp you are in and be sure the article you are choosing, after reading and rereading it, with note taking, is of that type. Are you going to use the article as a teaching platform to give an overview of the area, with the article serving as a jumping-off point, or are you focusing narrowly on the article? I prefer to learn about an area while I am researching a journal club presentation, and I enjoy sharing my new background knowledge with the group as a whole.

Recent reviews of journal clubs have highlighted the variability of these groups. Deenadayalan and colleagues (2008) conducted a systematic review of the literature to identify the systems and practices of an effective journal club. The aims of journal clubs included improving participants' reading habits and increasing skills in critical appraisal, knowledge of the current literature, research methods, and statistical analyses. The authors noted a wide variation in the amount of preparation expected, ranging from reading and studying the article beforehand to no preparation at all. The article could be chosen by group consensus or picked because it was relevant to a current program's curriculum or to a clinical area. Some journal clubs use a structured work sheet to note important data and its analysis.

Deenadayalan et al. (2008) reported that ten of twelve research articles that looked at the impact of journal club activities found that the journal club made a significant impact on one measured variable, such as knowledge of biostatistics and research design or critical appraisal skills, compared to a control activity, such as lectures or reading on one's own. Journal club format frequently included a designated journal club leader or a supervisor of journal club activities, who would often choose the paper to be presented. This person was usually a respected academic leader. Journal clubs usually meet monthly rather than weekly. Articles are frequently sent out ahead of time. As a result of this systematic review, Deenadayalan et al. concluded that, while attendance at journal clubs is a well-accepted practice, there is scant knowledge on the most effective way to conduct a journal club to gain the most educational value from it. A few of the articles reviewed described helping the journal club presenter initially choose an article. Deenadayalan et al. noted that an article that is relevant to the attendees sets the tone for a successful journal club. Participant preparation also helps to increase the probability of a "meaningful" discussion. Lunchtime journal clubs with food stimulated a higher attendance rate.

Hartzell et al. (2009) developed a resident-run journal club based on adult learning theory and compared it to their former journal club model to assess residents' attitudes and satisfaction with the new model. They note that journal clubs are often designed to stay current with medical literature and to achieve the requirements of the Accreditation Council for Graduate Medical Education for teaching critical reading skills and evidence-based medicine. Hartzell et al.'s paper describes the original format for their journal club as held once monthly. It focused on reviewing one article per session, under the guidance of an appointed faculty mentor who had expertise in epidemiology and clinical research and a senior teaching resident who was on a rotation to increase teaching skills. The article to be discussed was chosen by the resident, with minimal guidance, and then given out at the beginning of the journal club. House staff at the journal club was then divided into four groups, with each group focusing on one of the following parts of the article: introduction, methods, results, and the clinical implications. Most of the time was devoted to critical appraisal and biostatistics and much less to clinical significance. Given house staff dissatisfaction, a new model, based on an understanding of adult learning theory, was implemented.

Adult learning theory encourages learners to be more involved in planning the educational activity and selecting the curricular content. Learners then feel more comfortable expressing themselves. The new journal club had several goals: (1) run the club with faculty supervision, (2) review both current and landmark articles, (3) apply critical appraisal skills to the article review, (4) increase knowledge of biostatistics, (5) improve resident participation and attendance, (6) focus on the clinical significance of the articles, and (7) create a reference library of reviewed articles. The format for the club is a lunchtime meeting with free food and is forty-five minutes long. Two articles are presented, at twenty minutes each. The residents use Critical Appraisal Tool software (Oxford Centre for Evidenced-Based Medicine) to organize and streamline their presentations and to encourage maximum discussion. A survey, completed by 87.5 percent of the eligible internal medicine residents, identified the optimal characteristics of the journal club: it occurred at lunchtime, lasted an hour, and reviewed two articles at each session. The great majority felt that the club fostered their knowledge and that the articles were relevant to their patients. Ninety-two percent found that a subspecialist faculty at the journal club increased learning. Eighty-nine percent liked to have the articles beforehand. Only 39 percent of residents found the Critical Appraisal software helpful to their presentation, but the authors noted that if residents were given help with the software and became comfortable with it, their satisfaction increased. In their discussion, Hartzell et al. (2009) note that getting residents to engage in journal clubs is both important and challenging. They felt that the survey indicated that the new journal club model was well received compared to the old. Part of the success, Hartzell and his colleagues reasoned, was due to making the journal club an empowering process for the residents, teaching them a set of skills they could use on their own in the future when caring for patients, researching the literature, and assessing clinically relevant articles.

In summary, suggestions for success include: (1) using a structured tool–checklist to organize the article's analysis; (2) providing food; (3) reviewing only original research articles rather than clinical reviews or case reports; (4) setting a routine time and place for the meeting; (5) consistently teaching evidence-based medicine, statistical methods, and data analysis as part of the club's goals; (6) designating experts in the specialized area of the chosen journal club article at each meeting to foster discussion and provide timely answers to questions (Deenadayalan et al. 2008; Hartzell et al. 2009; Sidorov 1995).

Objective Structured Teaching Exercises

Teachers' and residents' performances can be measured in an analogous manner to those of medical students (Morrison 2002; Quirk 2006). In the objective structured teaching exercise (OSTE), the faculty member or resident interacts with a "standardized student" who has been taught to respond in a consistent manner. The faculty or resident being evaluated observes a student-patient interaction and is then expected to give feedback and explanations to the student based on his or her observations. It is the standardized student who completes the checklist to score the faculty or resident's teaching and feedback performance. OSTEs have been used to determine whether community preceptors are ready to teach in the ambulatory setting and to assess the effectiveness of faculty development interventions. They have also been used to assess residents' skills in clinical teaching. Elizabeth Morrison and colleagues have developed cases and rating scales that are made available free of charge to faculty wishing to use them for research or instruction (www.ucimc.netouch .com/contact.htm).

Wamsley et al.'s (2006) introductory workshop on OSTE is available online, with explanations, instructions, slides, cases, and rating scales (www.sgim.org/ userfiles/file/AMHandouts/AM06/handouts/WF06.pdf).

In an OSTE exercise on videotape of a student who was performing poorly in taking a patient's history, I watched the faculty member avoid giving appropriate feedback and direction, which would surely have increased the student's learning about the deficits of her performance. I also participated in an AAMC 2008 GEA/GSA miniworkshop on this methodology, entitled *Teachings, and Assessing Teaching Competencies Using OSTEs*, organized by Janet Hafler, EdD, and taught by Jenny Skolfield, MS, Laura K. Snydman, MD, Robert Trowbridge, MD, and Bob Bing-You, MD. As a faculty member, I had to give feedback on a less-than-adequate student history taken from a patient with back pain. I was keenly aware of how difficult and complex it is to give pithy, appropriate, and useful feedback on a subpar student performance. Bing-You and Trowbridge (2009) suggest that medical faculty may not be giving effective feedback because of inadequately developed metacognitive skills, such as reflection. Metacognition refers to the ability to think about one's thoughts and feelings and helps a learner know how well he or she is performing (Quirk 2006). Adequate metacognition or reflection is essential for feedback information to be properly translated and interpreted by learners. Bing-You and Trowbridge (2009) note that "effective feedback may require a mutual and trusting bidirectional negotiation process with give and take."

✌ TAKE-HOME POINTS
- Team-based learning permits one expert teacher effectively and dynamically to teach a large class in small groups by acting as a facilitator.
- 3S's—same problem, specific assignment, and simultaneous presentation—aid the effective use of groups.
- Team-based learning improves student attitudes toward learning, encourages team-building skills, and promotes active learning.
- No difference in objective scores on national tests has been noted as a result of team-based learning.
- Choose your journal club article carefully; it is easier to present "great" rather than "shoddy" research.
- Review the journal club article's statistical analyses early on with a full-fledged statistician; if the methods are flawed, the article may be fatally flawed—avoid it.
- Explain the importance of the article's research by giving some pertinent background information for those who are not knowledgeable about the area; your audience will then be on board to understand the point of your presentation.

- Consider visual aids, such as slides or a prepared blackboard presentation, to make the journal club presentation an effective educational experience.
- Send your journal club article to all who generally attend journal club ahead of time; the discussion will be better.
- Designate a faculty member as your journal club expert; be sure to formally invite this person to be at your journal club.

CHAPTER ELEVEN

Leading Others to Teach Well

- *What are the qualities I need to succeed as a leader?*
- *How do I run a successful teacher's meeting?*
- *How do I get noticed as a potential leader?*
- *How do I motivate teachers to do their best?*
- *Who will best help me to succeed?*
- *Are there resources to help me improve my educational leadership skills?*

The Qualities of Successful Leadership

Some leaders lead by persuasion; others by collegiality, collaboration, example, positive reinforcement, or focusing on a common goal. I classify my style of leadership as conscientious, collegial, collaborative, supportive, and goal oriented (Diamond, Gardiner, and Wheeler 2002; Ferren and Stanton 2004; Kaagan 1997). I avoid intimidation, shaming, autocracy, and negative reinforcement.

For each educational innovation, I recruit excellent teachers, who are outspoken and honest in their opinions. I look for loyalty to our common goal. I solicit their advice and frequently take it, even when it is different from my own. I am conscientious and have a plan that is well thought out; I am collegial when I respect other teachers' and administrators' abilities and advice. I am collaborative because I am willing to share credit with anyone who helps get the project off the ground. I am goal oriented and keep focused on winning great evaluations and prizes.

Educational leadership means convincing administrators as well as colleagues to buy into my ideas and to help me reach my vision (Diamond, Gardiner, and Wheeler 2002; Ferren and Stanton 2004; Kaagan 1997). It means listening to the administrator's feelings, concerns, and perception of the limitations regarding budget, personnel, and space. It means recognizing and respecting what boundaries the administrators set and what efforts they will expend to help. The boundaries may be the amount of time, money, space, resources, or personnel they allot to my project. The efforts may include creative and innovative ways of reaching our goal.

Table 11.1 lists components of effective leadership style.

How to Be an Effective Leader

Lead by example. Don't expect respect for your leadership skills if you are late, are disorganized in your plan and approach, or do not have a clear vision of where to go with your teaching efforts. If you are calling a meeting, this is your chance to shine as a leader, not to be a flop. Be alert to your reputation as a good leader. Other people's time is precious. Don't waste it with poorly prepared meetings that go nowhere. Put yourself in their place and try to feel how annoyed you would be if an hour-long meeting could have been summarized in one or two sentences.

The major preparation for a meeting comes from you, not your administrator. Each meeting should have a specific purpose, which can be achieved only when people meet face to face. This means that you need a plan that involves each person you call to this meeting. How do you do this? You ask questions that you want your committee to answer. Letting them know the questions beforehand is important for the meeting to succeed. Organize meetings in this way to respect your colleagues and to win their admiration for your planning and organizational skills. One or more of the committee members may one day recommend you for a promotion on the teacher-clinician ladder.

Table 11.1.   Components of Effective Leadership Style

1. Communicate a realistic vision of the final target
2. Obtain pertinent background information
3. Produce a step-by-step plan for how to reach the goal
4. Develop a checklist for covering the steps
5. Express a strong interest in hearing other opinions
6. Demonstrate a readiness to modify plans
7. Initiate the project as a collaborative effort
8. Give credit to those who contribute to success
9. Praise all forms of success
10. Have a sense of humor
11. Admit when you are wrong
12. Lead by example
13. Back down completely when you recognize that you are off base

Design the meeting so that each five-to-fifteen minute interval is allotted to a separate agenda item. Make the meeting move briskly, lingering only over the issues that you feel need discussion. Focus intently on topics that may have to do with future directions, unsettling news, or recent evaluations.

Send out your agenda several days in advance so that each person attending the meeting knows what is expected. Knowing the agenda also gives faculty members who were not planning to attend the meeting the option to change their minds. Go over the agenda the day before with your administrator, emphasizing the need for handouts to be printed and brought to the room by you or the administrator. Be careful of leaving the chore of providing handouts to someone else unless you have access to that person's office at the hour of the meeting and it is close to the meeting site.

If your administrator is coming from a distance or the meeting is at an early hour, you may wish to bring the handouts yourself. If the room is unfamiliar to your group, have the administrator post signs pointing the way in the lobby of the building and again as people step off the elevator. Treat your meeting members like honored guests, and they will reward you with their best opinions.

Successful leaders get things done by initiating the activity with enthusiasm, energy, an intelligent plan, and a keen sense of responsibility and accountability. They are "can do" people. Good leaders attract good colleagues to work with them because they have confidence in their colleagues' abilities. They delegate but also check on the status of the project periodically; they want no second guesses and no recriminations, and they do not want the project to flounder (Kaagen 1997).

Successful leadership means knowing when and how to go around a roadblock. A teacher who is a leader needs excellent communication, organizational, problem-solving, and motivational skills as well as creativity to make the teaching exercise come off as planned. If there is a problem, the teacher-leader steps in to solve it. He or she makes things happen, is the final arbiter and the bottom line.

Running a Worthwhile Tutor Meeting at the Preclinical Level

Many excellent teachers do not maximize their leadership capabilities when running an educational meeting. The meeting becomes a gabfest or gripe session rather than a place for learning, planning, creating, and doing. Table 11.2

Table 11.2.   Questions to Ask before Running an Educational Meeting

1. Why should tutors come to hear me when they might sleep later, prepare better, or organize their room and materials?
2. What do I have to offer that is worthwhile and may help tutors get ahead in teaching?
3. Will tutors gain new colleagues, new content knowledge, or teaching tips by coming?
4. Do I have a plan for each person to participate?
5. How far ahead should I send out the agenda?
6. How long should I wait to begin the meeting if few have shown up?
7. Did I remind tutors of the meeting the day before or the day of the meeting, or both, to maximize attendance?

lists questions to ask yourself before running an educational meeting. The following paragraphs will prepare you to run an efficient and effective meeting and demonstrate your leadership skills to peers.

The Mechanics

Organize a tutor meeting to the minute. Tutors are eager to get to their tutorial rooms. Have handouts ready to go. To get ready, be there half an hour or more before the meeting is to begin. Have your guest-experts take only five to ten minutes for their contributions or presentations, because you have a lot to accomplish in fifty minutes. This year, our tutor meetings were scheduled at 7–7:50 a.m. Almost all tutors showed up on time, despite the early hour. Never wait to start meetings; start at the time you indicated, even if few tutors are there, and you will gain the respect of those who came on time and those who were unavoidably late.

Get your own room ready to go before you leave to chair the tutor meeting. Setting up your room may take as much as an additional fifteen minutes. For a 7 a.m. meeting, I would plan on being at the medical school/hospital/conference center at 6:15, to be sure that all is ready to go smoothly. With travel time, this means waking up at 4:30 or 5 the day of these meetings. However, the early hour is worth it if your faculty shines during their individual sessions partly as a result of the teaching tips and content review you gave at the early-morning meeting.

We instituted a buddy system for new tutors in which each one is paired with an experienced tutor. The experienced tutor is frequently at the same hospital as the new tutor, which permits these teachers to get to know each other better as mentor and mentee. At the tutor meetings, we ask the buddy system tutors to sit with their "buddy" if possible so that they can more readily share experiences.

Preparation

- Remind tutors the day before a meeting, even if it is on the schedule.
- Make up an agenda with the course manager or administrator.
- Send the agenda out one or two days beforehand.
- Bring audiovisual material and make a reservation with the audiovisual department for the meeting time to be sure someone is there to turn on the projector and project slide sets.
- Schedule proper room size.
- Arrange coffee/tea for an early morning meeting.
- Erase the blackboard so that you can use it for your own diagrams.
- Have available an overhead projector or LCD projector and screen.
- Arrange parking for those who need it.

Agenda

- Have tutors make introductions, giving their name, hospital, and specialty interest. Include substitute tutors.
- Hold a round robin to discuss each tutor's group.
- Teach on the blackboard the current case content with concepts clearly spelled out. Focus at the end on the content for the beginning of the next week's case.
- Announce critical pieces of information, such as exam dates and venues, quiz questions and subsequent scores, and pathology laboratories.
- Buddy system: ask tutors to sit together to get to know each other.
- Preview slides for the week's tutorial.
- Preview content for the following week in a superficial manner, except for the first day of the tutorial, which should be covered in depth.
- Go over cross-cultural care experiences of each tutor and involve the cross-cultural care experts.
- Review closure schematics for the important content that may be confusing.

- Discuss student evaluations, how to do them, and the necessary timeline.

Leader's Educational Objectives
Agenda for Weekly One-Hour Tutor Meeting during a Course

1. Tutors report on

    a. Tutorial group dynamics
    b. Student preparedness and participation
    c. Cross-cultural care discussions.

2. Review schematics and tutorial slides for current week's case.
3. Preview next week's case concepts, schematics, and slides.
4. Make tutors at the meeting feel their teaching is worthwhile.

For tutors to want to come to your meeting, you must make them feel worthwhile by giving them your undivided attention and the ability to speak about their own group and experiences at least once, but preferably twice during the fifty-minute meeting. Call on them in order around the table to have an equitable process. Let tutors know ahead of time that each will be called on to present his or her group at your faculty-development sessions. If you do not call on new tutors individually, you will risk the dominant and more seasoned tutors holding the floor and not leaving any time for the younger and more timid tutors to voice their opinions.

Tutors who come to the weekly tutorial meetings should feel that they have an advantage over those who did not come. If the meeting is viewed as a throwaway meeting, of little use, taking time for it early in the morning will be a source of discontent. Be prepared to defend each item on your agenda as essential if the tutor is to excel. In addition, put yourself in the tutor's shoes. Would you want to hear someone extol his or her agenda at 7 a.m. if it were not directly beneficial to you as a tutor?

Meetings should also give tutors information they can not easily get through announcements and e-mail messages, such as (1) how to do evaluations on Web-based survey instrument set up by the school, (2) review of the final exam and quizzes, so they know what questions are being asked, (3) students' positive comments about the tutors as a group and about the course as a whole, and (4) positive comments made about their individual performance as a tutor.

It is far better for tutors to feel that they are working hard for a successful course than for an unsuccessful course. Only if negative feedback is truly pertinent to them, as tutors, should they hear it from the course director as they are about to go to tutor in a course. Tutors have usually lost a considerable amount of time and money by coming to teach for long hours with little recognition and often no pay. To list the course woes to them is inappropriate and usually discourages them. The course's ratings can change dramatically up until the last hour of the course. Why unsettle your tutors by musing out loud on the vagaries of student responses, which are not set in stone and could change significantly in a day or two?

Run the tutor meeting like the television show *Washington Week,* as a fast-paced forum for tutors' views and a review session for essential materials, visuals, tutoring attitudes, and pearls of wisdom regarding the quiet or dominant student.

Supporting Other Teachers' Excellence

In 1997, a group of teachers, Sanjiv Chopra, MD, Suzanne Rose, MD, MSEd, Harland Winter, MD, and I, who were members of the Education Committee of the American Gastroenterological Association, decided that we wanted to demonstrate a problem-based learning style of teaching at our annual meeting. We put in a proposal and received approval from the association to showcase problem-based learning luncheons to teach other teachers this methodology. I volunteered to organize this teaching activity on an annual basis. Over the past years, the luncheons have consistently garnered outstanding ratings, despite new teachers joining and others leaving the roster. How do I lead this educational activity to a successful conclusion each year? I motivate each of the problem-based discussion teachers by my energy, enthusiasm, and respect for them and their unique talents. I am clear, fair, and flexible in my planning. I personally phone each teacher each year to remind him or her of the details of the method. I provide examples of the materials and handouts on problem-based learning created by Chopra and Rose, and I invite each teacher to be part of a terrific team that has demonstrated a winning track record. If a teacher receives less than stellar ratings, we go over why. The teacher decides what needs to be changed for the following year. I support the changes.

My philosophy is that any teacher who wants to succeed can, if he or she is shown how (Ramani 2006). Medical teachers are busy. Unless you give instructional tips for teaching to each teacher in your teaching group, you risk their failing at the teaching assignment. Don't be afraid to pamper and to provide for your teachers. Help the people you are leading to succeed through a comprehensive approach to faculty development (Wilkerson and Irby 1998). Hope that they surpass you. This is the mark of an excellent leader and teacher of teachers.

Encouraging people to teach well is an empty phrase unless backed up by the reality of showing them how to teach well and providing them with the tools to succeed. I give teachers the opportunity to improve, and I stand by them while they try. One or even two poor performances are not sufficient to take a teacher off my teaching roster if the person expresses the desire to improve the teaching or asks for help.

One of my happiest moments as a teacher occurred when tutors in the gastrointestinal pathophysiology course received the highest number of award certificates for achieving a perfect overall teaching score as a tutor compared to tutors in the other preclinical courses. After we did well for three years in a row, I knew that I was doing something right, but what? The winning combination is confidence in each teacher, high expectations, clear instructions, and comprehensive teaching materials, involvement in the teaching process, and stimulating faculty-development sessions. This is good leadership in action.

Being Noticed as a Potential Leader

Do a great job at whatever you are asked to teach and even a curmudgeonly professor will notice you. Be organized, knowledgeable, enthusiastic, energetic, and clear in your instructions. Don't hesitate to make constructive criticisms. You may be given a leadership position when one opens up. Alternatively, a new position will be created for you. If your supervisors and supporters do not feel you are ready for a leadership position, they may give you an apprentice position, in which you can learn the ropes. This proving ground will groom you for the job you want, but it may also groom you for other positions when they become available. Remember that medical teachers are generally thrilled to have new faculty, resident, or fellow teachers. These new teachers bring creative ideas, high energy, questions, and new ways of doing things. They keep the more senior teachers on their toes and provide a challenge. Teachers welcome others who wish to follow in their footsteps as leaders. All directors know that eventually they will need to relinquish their positions of leadership. Most prefer that the person who replaces them share their vision. Be helpful to a course or clerkship director, and you and he or she may both be happy with the outcome. Don't act as if you'd like to replace the director right there and then. Instead, pay your dues by climbing the ladder to teacher success.

Common ways of rising to a leadership position include: (1) doing a great job at a starter position, with enthusiasm and energy, (2) offering constructive criticism to improve the program you taught in and volunteering to help make your suggested changes, and (3) telling the director that you have an idea for an innovative teaching session, class, seminar, rounds, or journal club, which you believe you can make successful if given the opportunity.

Leadership Positions for Medical Teachers

Opportunities for leadership abound in medicine. Top leadership positions in medical teaching have titles such as dean of education, dean of medical education, dean of curriculum, dean of continuing medical education, dean of assessment, dean of faculty development, vice-chair for medical education, and vice-president for faculty development programs. Other important positions include directors of preclinical major courses; clinical clerkship directors; directors of patient-doctor introductory courses in the first, second, third, and fourth years; directors of fellowship programs; directors of residency programs; directors of student advising and student remediation. Leadership positions extend to individual course directors in the preclinical year courses (I am director for the gastrointestinal pathophysiology course); individual courses in the clinical years, such as a radiology, cardiology, or EKG course; director of journal clubs; director of invited lecture series or summer lecture series; director of grand rounds; director of physical diagnosis rounds; director of a hospital conference, such as morbidity and mortality; director of a specialty conference, such as a surgical complications conference or a cancer board conference, on a weekly or monthly basis. Moderators at continuing education courses and moderators at a national meeting research forum, symposium, breakout session, or problem-based learning sessions are also considered important leadership positions.

The possibilities are endless. If this is the case, strongly consider creating a new position by filling a need or a void in education that you have perceived. Make sure you do a great job during your first year at your new position to put to rest any qualms or criticisms others may have concerning a new conference or teaching series. Attend an excellent course giving you leadership skills, such as Harvard Macy Institute's Program on Leading Innovations in Health Care and Education (Harvard_Macy@hms.harvard.edu), run by Elizabeth Armstrong, PhD, and Clay Christensen, MBA, DBA (Friedrich 2002), the year-long Teaching Scholars Program for Educators in the Health Sciences at McGill University (Steinert et al. 2003), the Medical Education Scholars Program (MESP), also a one-year program (Gruppen et al. 2003), or the University of Washington's leadership development program (Robins, Ambrozy, and Pinsky 2006).

Every bit of your background counts toward gaining a leadership position. If you were a chief resident, or taught a class or patient-doctor course as a resident or medical student, or were part of a teaching corps or tutored other students, then make note of these prior experiences on your curriculum vitae. Your knowledge and experience may be what sets you apart from other candidates for a leadership position. If you have a master's degree in education or have taken education courses, seminars, or continuing education courses, make sure your boss knows of your firm commitment to being a medical educator. Acquire skills, if you do not have them, by taking courses or getting an advanced degree.

Start climbing the ladder by volunteering for even the lowest-level position. Do an outstanding job without complaining. Get things done well that others consider drudgery. Offer constructive criticism that is well thought out. Consider writing a list of recommendations that you send to the director as a way of showing your interest and enthusiasm for improving the teaching exercise. Most course or clerkship directors are glad to receive frank and honest appraisals of what could be better organized, better taught, or better addressed. They may ask you to help them improve what you have constructively criticized.

Surround yourself with admirable people who are as good as or better than you are. Pick loyal, trustworthy lieutenants. Avoid sycophants. Get straight shooters who tell you if you are on the wrong track. Find people who are willing to push you ahead, not keep you behind. Loyal, hard-working, smart, and honest administrators are essential. Part of your success in academic life will be determined by your ability to motivate not only your fellow teachers but also your support staff to do their best (Covey 1989, 2004). Choose flexible, interested, energetic, ambitious, and enthusiastic helpers, who will respond to your vision with respect and enthusiasm. In return, be kind and generous. You need to make each secretary or administrator an integral and important part of the teaching team by creating a successful team atmosphere and including them in the decision making.

Your administrators' suggestions, corrections, and organizational skills will make the difference between excellence and mediocrity. Their attitude toward other teachers will gain or lose colleagues for you. No teacher wants to be put down by your administrator or reprimanded or treated in a brusque or patronizing manner. Recruiting teachers requires you to have a pleasant and enthusiastic voice on the other end of the phone. You want someone who knows exactly how to make the potential teacher welcome and at ease. Pick people for their pleasantness, kindness, and loyalty first, and then for their organizational skills. With warm personal qualities in your administrator, who is the face of your course, your ability to rise on the ladder by recruiting and leading others will be great. However, you will be severely limited in your ability to rise by efficient but unpleasant, bulldog personnel. Those surrounding you count as the translators of your vision. Make sure your supporters buy into your vision and are willing to work hard to transmit it to others who may call or ask. Otherwise, they may undermine your efforts in ways, however subtle, that lead to failure rather than success. Rid yourself of a disloyal worker who disparages you to your face or behind your back. The next act of disloyalty may cost you your respect in the academic community and your chances of success.

Fulfilling Your Clinical Practice Obligations While You Teach

As a clinical teacher, you are dependent on your administrator as a first-line stand-in for you when you are heavily involved in teaching or leading courses. Keeping your clinical practice going smoothly while you are teaching is crucial. You need an administrator who listens to your patients and expertly fields the calls, triaging them appropriately. Never try to teach and leave your beeper or pager on. This shows a lack of clinical and leadership savvy. You did not delegate to someone else your responsibilities ahead of time when you knew you could not be in two places at once. To teach effectively, you must free your mind from clinical messages and details of care that will intrude on your focus and your effectiveness. Each of my three clinical administrators over the past fifteen years has been a big part of my successfully combining clinical and teaching work. I rely on my administrator to make the initial determination of whether the covering physician needs to be called immediately for a particular patient problem while I am teaching or whether I can return the patient's call later in the day, when the teaching is finished.

I frequently hear the complaint that a doctor's clinical administrator is mean and curt while the doctor is nice and pleasant to the patient. You and your administrator should speak with the same voice, same tone, same conscientiousness, and same pleasantness. I model the tone of my voice and my patience on the phone for my clinical administrator by sitting next to her and taking some calls so that she sees how I approach a difficult or demanding patient. Don't tolerate less than outstanding clinical administrative skills. You will not be able to teach or lead with the focus and peaceful mind you need if your clinical life is made even more complicated and frustrating by a rude administrator or an administrator who takes messages with inadequate data for you to complete the task when you return from teaching and the administrator has gone for the day. Encourage your administrator to anticipate problems and reward her or him for bringing patient's problems to your attention before they fester and cause harm.

Sharing Leadership Responsibilities: Pros and Cons

I became the sole course director after running the pathophysiology course for one year as part of a triumvirate. Having three co-course directors did not work out. After this experience, I sent a letter to the overall course director explaining my plan for changes to address the medical students' complaints and was given the job. I enjoy being sole course director because I can make course changes relatively quickly when things are going wrong. One day, my supervisor asked if I would agree to take on a junior teacher as co-director. Given my past experience with multiple directors, I said no to this proposal even though the person being recommended would have added new talents and energy. My persuasive explanation and my excellent course evaluations were sufficient to squelch this proposal for joint leadership.

What are the pros and cons of being a co-director rather than a sole director?

The pros are that the workload is divided and is more manageable, and the skills of the other teacher are often complimentary to yours, giving rise to a better overall set of skills. If you cannot be at a particular meeting, the other person may be able to be there, he or she will be able to recruit new teachers whom you do not know from his or her circle of acquaintances, and he or she can be a sounding board for new ideas. The cons are that it is hard to attain recognition for teaching even if you are excellent. Sharing the limelight may make it difficult to be given full credit for your portion of the work. Administrators and other personnel may find it easier to reach or work with one of you, thereby excluding the other from some of the day-to-day activities. Think carefully about accepting a partner in teaching; once the partner is on board, it is difficult, if not impossible, to go back on the bargain, which may be a bad one for your career advancement but a good one for the new arrival's career advancement.

Planning for Your Replacement

Keep looking for new talent to replace you. Groom others in your leadership skills and management style so that when you are ready to give up your leadership position, you will have others filling your shoes capably. Recognize that you may have little to do with choosing who is to replace you. Politics may enter into the decision if more than one teaching hospital seeks visibility at the medical school. It may be time for a new hospital group or department to take over the teaching position you are vacating if teaching responsibilities are to be fairly allocated. Prepare for your supervisor a list of those people you believe would do your job as well as or better than you. Indicate on the list your top three or four choices and the reasons. Even if no one on your list is given the position, you will have had a chance to influence the decision.

In an Instant, Everything Can Change

A few weeks ago, while driving into work, I noticed a new billboard saying, "In an instant, everything can change." This is true. In my mind, I compare being a course director to being a sports figure, whose ratings can change in a minute. I have taught you how to be a hero in teaching by using a framework. I have not discussed how easy it is to change from being a hero to being a dud.

At the end of a course that went extremely well, I made a tactical error while proctoring the final exam in a large auditorium. I demanded that I be able to see each and every student. Some students wanted to take their exams in seats, or on the floor, where they were partly hidden from view. The entire class became incensed. I could feel their anger, but I foolishly dug in my heels even though I sensed that I was in the wrong. In their view, I mistrusted all of them. Subsequently, the students' anonymous course evaluations went into unpleasant detail concerning their disappointment with me. This incident had wiped out their good feelings about me as a course director. The overall course ratings suffered significant damage as a result, and it took years to restore my reputation as a fair and honorable teacher. The lesson is to think carefully about every statement you make to the class, to medical students, and to learners. Gauge and anticipate the effect your comments may have. When in doubt about what to do, ask other teachers or people whom you trust to be honest with you.

✑ TAKE-HOME POINTS

- Persuade others to buy in to your vision through open communication.
- Be flexible and willing to change.
- Surround yourself with the best teachers.
- Credit others for their part in the project's success.
- Ask for expert opinions and take some for a trial run.
- Admit when you are wrong and avoid repeating the error.
- Lead by example, with well-organized and well-rehearsed meeting plans and agendas.
- Be hungry to rise and do a superb job to get there.
- Don't tolerate disloyalty or incompetence in your administrator or colleagues.
- Choose a conscientious clinical secretary who creates a peaceful and organized haven for patients.
- Consider all the pros and cons of taking on a teaching partner before you say yes; afterward, it may be too late.
- Weigh carefully statements to the whole class; some may work against your efforts to create the optimal learning atmosphere.

CHAPTER TWELVE

Recognition, Rewards, Awards, and Prizes

- ✂ *How do I improve my visibility and obtain recognition for teaching?*
- ✂ *What is a teacher's portfolio, and how do I keep it?*
- ✂ *How do I increase the probability of my receiving awards and prizes?*
- ✂ *May I nominate myself for a national or regional award?*

How to Obtain Recognition for Teaching

Knowledge of the process of moving up the teaching ladder toward recognition, rewards, awards, prizes, and promotion is the key to arriving at your career goals. Think of sprinters or swimmers who in high school set their eyes on the Olympic gold medal. Intense planning, preparation, and arduous work are essential for success in the four, eight, or twelve years that it may take to accomplish their goal. Academic medicine is no different. Acceptance and incorporation of guidelines, rules, tips, and coaching by those who have a track record of winning are crucial to understanding how to accomplish your goals and to achieving them.

Papp, Aucott, and Aron (2001) advocated greater rewards and recognition for clinical teachers in medicine as a means of retaining teachers. They recommend monetary support, along with strategies to advance careers through the clinician-educator track. Lowenstein, Fernandez, and Crane (2007) noted that in a survey of faculty members who were considering leaving academic medical centers, faculty believed that departments did not reward high-quality teaching and excellent clinical work. Establishing the clinician-educator track for promotion at medical schools has been one method of remedying this problem.

Preclinical teachers receive recognition for their teaching skills and scholarship through learner evaluations, peer evaluations, teaching awards, and objective measures such as their students' OSCE scores and USMLE, Step 1 and Step 2, scores (Simpson and Fincher 1999). A large audience may observe preclinical teachers' prowess through videotaped lectures and direct observation by expert teachers. Clinical teachers receive recognition through resident and student evaluations, peer evaluations, teaching awards, and residency and fellowship placement.

More recognition is given to directors of all types—preclinical or clinical course directors, hospital-based clerkship directors, residency and fellowship directors—than to other medical teachers. Because of their visibility, importance, and name recognition to a large audience of students, residents, and fellows, as well as other peer teachers, advisors, and administrators, course directors will more frequently be thought of and be in line to win awards and prizes than all the worthy teachers who are teaching alongside them. Levinson and Rubenstein (2000) cautioned that some excellent and effective teachers may not win teaching awards while popular teachers may. This makes the significance of awards for teaching more difficult to interpret.

If you want to be a course or clerkship director, tell pertinent people—the director of the first- or second-year curriculum, the dean of education, the dean of the medical school, the divisional chief of your department—of your interest in such a position. Tell them that you know you would do a great job and ask how you should go about gaining the position. Honesty is the best policy in trying to rise on the teaching ladder. Because many medical faculty members are too busy with clinical responsibilities, research projects, or other administrative efforts to take on a major teaching assignment, it is a relief for those in charge to receive an enthusiastic endorsement of teaching and of a commitment to helping improve the current state of teaching at all levels. Let the current course, clerkship, residency, or fellowship director know that you are eager to help in any way possible and to take on any teaching assignment they have a vacancy for. You never know when this person will decide to call it quits or move up the ladder or receive a research grant for another project. It is worth getting out the message that you are interested in larger teaching responsibilities and a leadership position and showing that you will take on lowly assignments to learn the ropes.

Course director and clerkship director positions are often held for five to ten years or longer if the director is accomplished and effective. However, I have seen these positions open up overnight as research grants, family ties, or poor evaluations change things rapidly and unexpectedly. If you have been teaching in this area, the vacancy may go to you, so know the terrain of the course, gain some experience in what you wish to pursue at the lower levels, do your best, even at menial tasks, and you may be perceived as a known, excellent commodity for the position when the time comes for change.

Even if you are not given a course or clerkship director position, you will often be remembered for the next leadership position in teaching that comes along. This "consolation prize" position may turn out to be a helpful career boost and may lead to even better future opportunities. I recommend taking what is offered and, like Rumpelstiltskin, spinning straw into gold. Some visibility is better than no visibility if you wish to succeed in teaching as a major part of your medical career.

Course directors usually receive some monetary compensation or salary for their efforts. Even small amounts of medical school or hospital moneys make your divisional or department chairman happier when you cut back on your clinical duties to teach.

If no course or clerkship director position or alternative leadership position is available, do the best and most enthusiastic and creative teaching you can do at the lower levels and hope for future recognition from students and peer faculty for your contributions. This will usually lead to higher-level responsibilities, with more recognition, over time.

Eventually, if you continue to receive outstanding evaluations for your teaching, you will be recognized by a reward such as a plum committee assignment or a prize. Relentless persistence and meticulous attention to achieving teaching goals are essential to reaching your goal of increased recognition.

If the system at your current institution is not conducive to your rise as a medical teacher, you may need to move to another institution, where the path is clearer for you to succeed. Be sure to have a signed contract with a designated medical education leadership position and promotion before you jump ship; you don't want to be disappointed again at the next institution.

Medical Teacher's Portfolio

Davis and Ponnamperuma (2005a, 348) write that teaching portfolios should be "self-portraits of teachers, providing vivid representations of themselves." Keep a detailed record (portfolio) of a broad range of educational scholarship and teaching activities, including all grades, evaluations, feedback, and self-reflections on teaching. Hafler and Lovejoy (2000) encourage separating the array of educational contributions into local, regional, and national levels at all ranks for promotion, while Dr. Patricia Thomas, at the Johns Hopkins University Medical School (http://deptmed.med.som.jhmi.edu/faculty/body11 .html), recommends that you document the diversity of the audiences you teach and the array of teaching methods that you use in your courses, workshops, and teaching exercises. In your CV, list which teaching activities refer to medical student, resident, faculty, and community audiences.

At the Medical College of Wisconsin, Beecher and colleagues established ten categories for documentation of teaching scholarship (www.mcw.edu/dis play/docid2546.htm). This organizational framework will help put your teaching activities into a format for eventual promotion. It also provides you with a method for reflecting on your teaching philosophy and career goals. The ten categories in the system, with slight modification, are:

1. Philosophy of Education: Personal theory of learning and teaching
2. Curriculum Development: Design, development, and evaluation of curricula/programs by peers and students
3. Teaching Skills: Documentation of teaching by target audience (medical students, residents, faculty, or community physicians), year, and topic
4. Learner Assessment: Construction and implementation of examinations/methods of assessment
5. Adviser: Lists of formal and informal advisees
6. Educational Administration: Leadership and management in education
7. Educational Scholarship: Research, publications, and presentations
8. Continuing Education: Evidence of growing knowledge and skills as an educator
9. Honors and Awards: Recognition by peers and students
10. Long-Term Goals: Reflection on portfolio and future plans

Subsequently, Beecher et al. (1997) showed that preparing the educator's portfolio stimulates reflection and promotes faculty development.

Rewards
Rarely are the monetary rewards of being a clerkship or course director sufficient to make up for the time spent teaching and doing administrative work for the course, clerkship, or residency/fellowship program. In addition, money

may be given to the chair of your department or division, in partial compensation for the time you spend developing curriculum and faculty, rather than to you as direct salary or to your chairperson as salary.

Be grateful for all monetary rewards, however paltry, because your department may be willing to let you buy out clinical time with the revenues from teaching in order to cut your clinical load. It is essential to use this time freed up from clinical responsibilities to create a course curriculum, faculty development program, or new organizational plans for teaching.

Visibility is the reward for preclinical and clinical clerkship and course director teachers. Without this, it is hard to gain recognition for future awards, prizes, and promotions.

Another reward is being put on a faculty committee for curriculum development or a new teaching project. These committees permit you to meet other faculty members, from whom you can learn and share ideas for fruitful collaborations and innovations.

It is uncommon, but not impossible, to receive a salary raise for excellent teaching. Generally, medical teachers' salaries are significantly lower than those of others in the department unless a medical educator has major administrative responsibilities for teaching, as head of an academy, dean of medical education at a medical school, or head of a teaching institute, where a portion of this person's salary may come for performing administrative tasks and educational initiatives.

Grants and teaching fellowships are available to help further your research into creating curricula or designing new faculty development programs, multimedia Web sites, or tutorial formats. Having visibility helps you in the competition for these funds.

Awards

Medical schools generally recognize excellent teachers with awards and annual award ceremonies. Awards usually come with a plaque, framed certificate, and statement of the comments accompanying the nomination, whereas a prize usually indicates that a small monetary reward also accompanies the certificate or plaque. Both are great ways to gain recognition for your efforts, because these awards are usually published in the medical school or hospital news, along with photographs and accolades. Earn as many awards and prizes as possible to show sustained excellence in teaching over a prolonged period of time.

Being in the right place at the right time is an important key to obtaining many of these awards. If the class has just had several poor lecturers, you may benefit from being a good lecturer. Similarly, if the tutorial group has been frustrated in their learning by a prior tutor who talked excessively or did not have sufficient content expertise or confidence, you may benefit if you are efficient and effective in your discussion of complex concepts with this same group. Listen carefully to all negative criticisms of those who have gone before you and take the criticisms seriously if you wish to succeed where others have failed. Try not to repeat mistakes in teaching. Never ignore criticism of a teaching session or become defensive. Do something about changing your teaching offering, whether lecture, small group, seminar, tutorial, or laboratory exercise. Find out what is driving the criticism (such as a good educational offering at the wrong time), and try to address this issue.

Nominations for teaching awards and prizes frequently come from unlikely quarters. The least assuming, quiet student rather than the dominant or brilliant leader of the group or class is generally the one who nominates you for awards.

All students, residents, and fellows are potential nominators. Be kind, pleasant, well prepared, and unflappable no matter what happens in class, tutorial, or small-group session. Your serene competence will give you extra points toward a nomination. Each person you teach may be responsible for your recognition and promotion. I have seen awards go to teachers who had only a fraction of the expected student group in their lecture or small group, but they gave such a memorable, powerful, and polished presentation that they were applauded by this small group, who went on to nominate them for an award.

Learners who rave to your face about your great teaching are generally not the ones writing the nominations. Rather, having given you the praise to your face, these students, residents, or fellows often do not sit down to write the nomination. Other learners, who are reticent to approach you with praise, may be the ones submitting a letter on your behalf to the nominating committee. If no one rushes up to compliment you, do not despair. You may still win an award if you have done an excellent job.

Nominate yourself for teaching or educational awards at the regional or national level. No one but you really knows your contributions and the impact they have made. Toot your own horn. You will be glad you did. Let your chair know that you are writing the nominating letter for yourself and would appreciate his or her signing it. If at first you do not succeed with a national or regional recognition award, try again the next year. Most organizations have a list of perennial nominees. Eventually some of these people will win the award. It does not matter how many times you have been proposed for the award. Winning the award could change your career prospects considerably, so try again, if you are qualified.

Find out who is receiving the awards and why the awards are being given. Go to the teaching award ceremonies. Nominating letters or excerpts of nominations will be read during the ceremony extolling the virtues of the awardees. Nomination letters give a good picture of why the award is being given and what the judging committee is looking for in awarding prizes and awards. Is it humanism? Is it content expertise? Is it the ability to inspire through words? Is it the organizational abilities shown in directing a course or clerkship? Is it creative exercises that encourage students to love medicine? Is it clarity in the explanation of complex concepts or something else? What is it? To improve, you will need to seek role models among the pantheon of repeat award winners to dissect the expertise, content presentation, personality traits, and organizational skills that permit them to win year after year or at least be nominated multiple times.

Once you recognize who the great teachers are, watch their teaching videos, which are generally available online at your medical school. Ask to see the great teachers' course syllabi, watch them give grand rounds, a seminar, or a subspecialty conference. What are they doing differently from you? How does their method inspire students, peers? How do they present themselves, their content? What is the logic of the course organization? What are the objectives of their course? How does the syllabus meet the objectives?

Copy great teachers' methods, demeanor, personality, and organizational skills. Read books on good teaching. Great teachers are labeled great so the rest of us can try to emulate them. They are doing something right. Do not be afraid to copy them.

Your audience will not change its ideal of great teaching. To earn the desired awards and prizes and the name recognition that goes with them, you must change your style, content, preparedness, delivery, organizational efforts, or philosophy.

✖ TEACHING TIPS

1. **Learn from and copy "great" teachers.**
2. **Because awards, prizes, and recognition go most readily to course and**

clerkship directors, try to gain one of these positions, even if you have to ask to be appointed.

3. Nomination letters for awards and prizes frequently come from quiet, un-obtrusive students, residents, or fellows. Be your best with every learner.

✣ TAKE-HOME POINTS

- Win every award you can. The number of awards counts but does not guarantee promotion at the top ranks.
- Teaching awards or prizes will not guarantee the rank of full professor; publications and national and international visibility will.

CHAPTER THIRTEEN

What to Do When Time Does Not Permit Optimal Preparation for a Teaching Assignment

- *Who can help you prepare?*
- *Whom should you call?*
- *What tools do you have at your disposal?*
- *How can you successfully anticipate this problem?*
- *Should you ever refuse an assignment?*
- *Can you change the assignment to better suit your talents?*

Facing the Unknown: Attending Physician and Consult Responsibilities

As an attending physician on medicine or surgery or as a consult attending physician on a specialty service, you will frequently be asked questions that you may have only a vague idea how to answer. In these cases, sick inpatients, the house staff and attending team, and the family await your response. To answer the questions posed in the consult, you will immediately go to the literature to find the answer or consult someone who is an expert in the area. Your quick search of the literature and development of an immediate plan of action for diagnosis and management is essential to good medical practice. Communicating your knowledge and decision-making clearly, quickly, and well is the hallmark of the outstanding consultant, who moves heaven and earth to obtain the best answer as quickly as possible for the patient, the family members, and the team. However, being a great and respected consultant is not what the rest of this chapter discusses. Rather, it focuses on the nonemergency aspects of being a teaching attending, particularly when you are asked to speak at a conference about a topic about which you know little.

The Dreaded Last-Minute Teaching Assignment

Occasionally, a medical teacher is asked to comment on something about which he or she knows little for a teaching session less than an hour or two away or early the next morning. You can approach this assignment as: (1) an opportunity to learn quickly about a subject you are unfamiliar with; (2) a "hot potato" to be passed along to someone else; or (3) a chance to practice your ability to say, "No, I am unable to do this at present, but would be happy to comply with your request at another date and time." Frequently, if you choose 2 or 3, you will be asked to identify and recruit your own replacement for the assignment. The time you spend getting a replacement, explaining to the replacement why you cannot do the assignment, and thanking him or her profusely for doing the assignment may begin to equal the amount of time you would need to speak on the topic yourself. If time is not the issue, but expertise is, find a replacement. If, on the other hand, the reason you cannot drop everything to prepare is that you are in the midst of a patient crisis or up against a grant deadline, then be careful of volunteering to obtain a replacement. Suggest names, but let the inviter do the calling.

A medical teacher who has a reputation for being excellent cannot turn in a poor performance without repercussions. Medicine is only too happy to topple teachers, researchers, and clinicians who seem to have overstepped their bounds or been given too much praise. Your reputation is yours to lose; hang on to it. Be careful not to accept an assignment beyond your scope or available time.

Whom to Turn to for Help

When faced with a last-minute assignment on something about which I know little, yet do not feel I can pass along to someone else or postpone, I turn to the following people for help: (1) a librarian, (2) a media specialist, (3) my practice administrator, (4) a fellow, (5) an expert. I have used the following steps to achieve moderate success with these difficult assignments.

First, I push the panic button, pick up the phone, and call the librarian for help to find the best articles pronto (Holst et al. 2009). The hospital and medical school librarians know me well from past interactions involving teaching, publication, and research. I run to the library to read the latest textbooks and pick up the articles from the librarian to speed-read. I quickly make a decision regarding my objectives, emphasis, angle, and take-home message. I develop a series of questions to ask out loud to provide a framework for the audience to logically structure the learning.

Second, I call my media specialist and ask if she or one of her group is willing to develop a slide set from algorithms, diagrams, tables, or figures that I or the librarian sends to her while I continue to try to digest the literature. If the answer is no, I try to develop the slide set myself or go without visuals and use copies of the best papers as handouts for the presentation. I plan to use a blackboard or whiteboard for explanations, lists, or diagrams if one or the other is in the room where I will be teaching.

Third, I call my practice administrator to obtain the medical record numbers of patients I have seen who have the condition under discussion. I look at the charts of these patients to find the consultants who saw or operated on the patients. I may be able to quickly create a problem-based learning vignette, which can be photocopied and serve as the jumping-off point for discussion and questions.

Fourth, I ask my specialty fellow for help with the presentation, especially if I know that he or she has had in-depth exposure, through a rotation on a relevant specialty service or through a research project, to the problem I am to discuss.

Fifth, I call an expert consultant and ask if he or she is willing to come with me to discuss the problem. If not, I ask the expert consultant to give me a five-minute explanation, on the phone, of the state of the art of this topic, the best diagnostic methods, and the current therapies.

By the time I finish with one or more of the steps, I have an idea of what I will say, how I will say it, and how I wish to interact with the audience.

Tools That Can Help

Pub Med, Google, and Paper Chase help me locate clinical and research articles. In addition, I like to skim through the latest editions of standard medicine textbooks and specialty textbooks to obtain an overview of the field before narrowing my focus. I am careful to set time limits for myself so that I do not get too wrapped up in reading. I still need to decide on objectives, synthesize, distill, devise a summary, and create take-away points. I watch my clock carefully and apportion my time from the beginning. I stick to my schedule to be ready to teach the new subject on time with handouts, a slide set, or at the minimum, a distillation, summary, and take-home points.

Anticipating the Problem

Box up your vignettes, cases, best x-rays, slide sets, and endoscopic photos, and have them ready as canned, interesting cases. I keep mine in one place. How does this help? It helps when one of the consults you were scheduled to see and discuss is not on the floor when you go to see him or her but is stuck in x-ray or the cardiac echo lab. You and your team are left with follow-up cases to discuss. A canned or boxed case with objectives, visuals, and a great punch line will do wonders for otherwise tedious rounds. Have the group members face one another in a circle and pass out the collated pages of a canned case. Ask them to talk to each other and solve the complex problem. By the time they finish, the consult patient will be on the floor and you will have received accolades for not letting rounds be boring or for not canceling the teaching part of rounds.

In your boxed set of cases, you may have something that bears on the topic you are being asked to discuss on the fly. Use it, even if it is peripheral. Is it a great film, pathology specimen, unusual history of physical finding, or unusual set of lab data? As long as you clarify what point you are emphasizing, go for a bold visual stroke; it creates a memorable image, good will, and excitement about medicine in your audience.

Refusing the Assignment

Although refusing the assignment sounds impolitic to do, it may be the best decision for the reason mentioned above: your reputation. "Nothing ventured, nothing gained" does not apply here. What does apply is that looking unprepared, ill read, or apologetic about the superficial level of your knowledge is hard for your audience to forget. My advice is to postpone rather than perform at a low level.

Using Sleight of Hand

You can maintain your reputation for teaching excellence when faced with a subject you know you do not know by using substitution. Substitution may resemble a boardwalk shell game using sleight of hand, but I recommend trying it. What do I mean? Ask the person who has called, paged, or e-mailed you if you can substitute something you know a lot about, rather than something you know little about. Tell the person you have a great presentation you know the group would like to hear. Few faculty, fellows, or residents will refuse the substitution when you offer them a great talk on a silver platter, unless the topic you were asked to discuss is essential to the patient's management that day. Otherwise, tell them that you will be ready to discuss the original topic in a few days, buying time to research the topic properly and pull together a valuable teaching presentation. You will win points for your candor, enthusiasm, and willingness to learn.

Instead of a didactic presentation, suggest a bedside history or physical exam session. Use a patient whose diagnosis is based on a history or physical exam finding that was missed by all but the medical student or resident. Make it a mystery case for others on the team who do not know the final diagnosis. You can shine in this type of venue. Consider making up hypothetical cases to illustrate classic medical pitfalls in diagnosis and management; house staff teams enjoy hearing about mistakes and how to avoid them.

Tell the person who invited you that you would prefer to give the team of fellows, residents, and students helpful tips about career choices, interviewing dos and don'ts, and navigating the academic system. You acknowledge your past success with this perennially useful topic, while agreeing to discuss the complex new topic later in the week or the following week. Alternatively, suggest the names of the appropriate experts and, if you have time, ask them to give the talk instead of you.

Ask if your personal philosophy of patient care or your approach to the management of the difficult patient could be substituted as a memorable contribution to the training of future physicians.

Good Teaching Requires Preparation and Forethought

Teaching is not a curbside consult or an emergency opinion. Objectives, patient case, well-researched literature, excellent visuals, summary, and take-away points are time-consuming to create. Suggest that you need more time to prepare a teaching session. You will not regret it. If no leeway is possible, follow the steps above to ask others for help in quickly creating a worthwhile discussion of the topic.

✎ TEACHING TIPS
1. **Ask your hospital or medical school librarian for help.**
2. **Ask your media department to make a slide show of the material you send or bring to them; media services understand "crunch time."**

3. Request help from your secretary in retrieving cases and medical record numbers; create one-paragraph, powerful vignettes.
4. Use your fellows' knowledge of the latest literature; bring them into the limelight in return.
5. Guide your thinking about the subject after discussions with experts; bring them along if possible.
6. Deftly refuse an assignment or substitute, with permission, a subject and presentation you know well.

✂ TAKE-HOME POINTS

- Avoid damage to your reputation as an excellent teacher; it may be long lasting.
- Focus on what you know, unless you have time to research what you do not know.
- Be careful of volunteering to obtain a replacement if you have no time to do this.
- Give ample credit to all who help you; your reputation will increase.

CHAPTER FOURTEEN

Bringing an Educational Research Project to Completion

- What hypothesis am I trying to prove or disprove with this research project?
- What outcome or assessment measures will I use?
- How do I determine the order of the authors?
- How do I obtain approval from the Institutional Review Board?
- To what journals should I submit medical education research?
- Is submitting an abstract to an educational meeting worthwhile?

Overview of Publishing Educational Research Projects

The field of medical education is full of research opportunities. Each change in curriculum, new faculty development program, or innovative laboratory exercise lends itself to evaluation and assessment of outcome data. As in clinical or bench research, a clear hypothesis, experimental and control groups, end points for assessment, appropriate statistical analyses, and careful review of the background literature are standard requirements. In addition, medical schools and hospitals require informed consent from students and faculty who are used as subjects in research studies. Effectively navigating the institutional review boards of the medical school or hospital is essential. It is helpful to use a poster or oral presentation of your data to obtain advance constructive criticism and suggestions before submitting the research manuscript for publication.

I began my first educational research project, in June 2002, on a new method for tutorials that integrated three Harvard Business School teaching strategies into a problem-based second-year gastrointestinal pathophysiology tutorial. This project was given two crucial years of initial funding by the Academy at Harvard Medical School (Thibault, Neill, and Lowenstein 2003) so that I could complete the educational research with salary support for my time. The project was entitled "A faculty development program to train tutors to be discussion leaders rather than facilitators." The educational research paper was published almost five years later, in May 2007. I submitted the manuscript in 2006 to my first-choice journal, *Academic Medicine*; the paper required major revisions initially, as well as minor revisions later, before it was finally accepted for publication. I started my second educational research project, entitled "Integration of racial, cultural, ethnic, and socioeconomic factors into a gastrointestinal pathophysiology course," in October 2005. *Clinical Gastroenterology and Hepatology* published it in March 2009, three and a half years later. I am not advocating these long gestation periods for research projects, but it can take that long to collect data that are sufficiently strong, to write and submit the manuscript, wait for reviews, make the suggested revisions, obtain additional data, if needed, to finally see your work in print. Quinn and Rush (2009, 634) point out that "writing takes a lot of time. You must set aside uninterrupted time." Steinert et al. (2008) encouraged writing by faculty members in the area of medical education by having a workshop and ongoing peer writing-group to facilitate writing productivity.

If the first journal does not accept the article, keep trying other journals while changing the manuscript in accord with the criticisms received from the rejecting journal. Your research will likely eventually be accepted, but it may take several tries until a medical education journal or a specialty journal in your field (interested in publishing medical education articles) accepts your innovation. The latter was the case with my second article, in which gastroenterologists who teach pathophysiology recognized the utility of integrating cross-cultural care into a gastrointestinal pathophysiology course's tutorials. Getting published in the educational arena is every bit as competitive as getting published in the basic science or clinical realm. Because relatively few journals are devoted to medical and health education, acceptance rates are low, particularly at top journals, such as *Academic Medicine*. Online publication is another possibility, on the MedEd Portal Web site of the Association of American Medical Colleges (www.aamc.org/mededportal).

Where do you find ideas for research projects? Everything you do educationally is a potential research project. Research projects may be focused on the outcomes of whatever innovation you are planning in a course, curriculum, or clerkship. You can evaluate skills, performance, attitudes, and outcome measures (Chen, Bauchner, and Burstin 2004). All is fair game. The biggest stumbling block is recognizing that no research study is handed to you labeled as such but that everything you do to improve medical education is a possible research study.

Begin your research project with a question or a hypothesis. Develop a hypothesis—a straw man that you wish to shore up or knock down based on your observations as a teacher (Cook, Bordage, and Schmidt 2008). You may believe that one method of lecturing is preferable to another or that simulation laboratories can offer specific improvements in OSCE scores. Take your question or hypothesis and clarify and simplify it. Then begin to turn it into a research project by determining how you will answer your question. How will you test whether your hypothesis is valid? Will you make up a questionnaire, an evaluation form, a new curriculum, an OSCE, a simulation laboratory, a tutorial method, or a team-based learning project? What will you measure as an outcome? Will your study be descriptive and observational, or will it be focused on statistical analyses? Alternatively, consider basing your research on your prior teaching experiences, the observations you have made, and questions that have arisen as a result. You will undoubtedly have questions about the methodology used, the evaluations obtained, and interventions for the next time you teach. Try to answer these questions by designing a research project that is methodologically rigorous and capable of generating evidence of effectiveness and efficiency in the medical education innovation or intervention (Dauphinee and Wood-Dauphinee 2004).

Next, decide on the methodology that will answer your question or prove your hypothesis. Will a questionnaire provide the data set, or will you analyze a performance exam, national board scores, final examination scores, attitudinal surveys, or satisfaction indices? Who will help you? These are your collaborators. How will they help you? How will you as a research group divide up the work to be done? Who will be responsible for what? Establish a chain of command early to give organization and clarity to the hierarchy of your group. Someone must be in charge of the research effort. Will that be you or someone else? How often will your group meet to discuss your progress? How will you analyze the data that you collect? You will need a statistician if you do not feel comfortable doing the statistics yourself. Most medical schools have departments with medical educators and assessment groups who are familiar with doing the requisite statistical analyses. Statisticians are more than willing to weigh in on the initial design of the project so that the best data are collected most efficiently. The statistician is a valued member of any research team and likely the best member to point out potential deficiencies in data collection and management before the study starts.

Several medical educators have made pertinent observations about deficiencies in the field of medical education research and have suggested some options for improvement. Shea, Arnold, and Mann (2004) note that medical education research needs to study the relationships of educational programs to health outcomes. Regehr (2004) also suggests that in medical education research, communal efforts across programs are necessary to build knowledge and understanding rather than end up with an uncoordinated collection of data and information by medical education researchers working in isolation. Gruppen (2007) highlighted the technical issues in medical education research compared to basic science or clinical research, specifically, small sample size, lack of a true control group, difficulty of randomization, inadequate descriptions of study methods (so that replication can be attempted), and lack of the relevance of outcome measures between educational interventions and patient outcomes. Gruppen (2007, 335) recommends collaborative initiatives to address some of these problems, "for in numbers lies strength."

Authorship

Who will write up the study? Who will be first and who will be last author? I ask about authorship expectations at the first meeting of the research-project working group (Quinn and Rush 2009). Authors are not only those who write up the manuscript but also those who contribute to the intellectual content, who collect, generate, and analyze observational data or perform statistical analyses on quantitative data, who revise the manuscript, and who give significant suggestions and advice as to how to perform the study. Asking about authorship early on helps establish who is considering himself or herself the likely first author. This person is in charge of moving the study forward and of writing up the results. The person who writes the paper from start to finish is generally the first author, even if the idea for the project did not originate with him or her, because taking a paper through its writing and revision phases involves a major outlay of time, which frequently involves nights and weekends. If someone does all the data collection and analyses, but then leaves to go to another institution or is unable to write up the study for other reasons, he or she may still be first author, if the person who writes up the study agrees that this is the fair thing to do. Alternatively, the person who writes up the study may be first author and the one who did much of the work can be second author or the last author. Many journal citations list only the first three authors, so the first three authorship spots are important for visibility and career advancement. Theoretically, the author in the last spot gave important guidance, made crucial suggestions, asked the question that motivated the study, gave laboratory space, equipment, techniques, or personnel or other support to help complete the study. This senior (last) author is often well established and has a track record in the field of publications. Sometimes the senior author is given authorship as a sign of respect, when he or she had little to do with the design or day-to-day research. Does where you are in the lineup of authors matter? In trying for promotion, the number of papers for which you are either first, second, third, or last (senior) author does count, and the promotions committee takes note of your bibliography.

The position of corresponding author also takes on significance if the first author and corresponding author are not one and the same person. What is the corresponding author? The corresponding author is the person who will answer all questions from the journal editors regarding the manuscript, submit the conflict-of-interest forms and copyright transfer forms for everyone, and be responsible for sending out a reprint or the PDF file to those who request them. Frequently, the corresponding author, if not also the first author, is the last author, because the first author is leaving town, or has left the group for another university position, or is a fellow or junior faculty member who was not involved in all phases of the study or who does not wish to have the possible burden of being responsible for reprint requests or answering questions that arise during the journal submission process. The last author sometimes asks to be the corresponding author as a way of exerting control over the progress of the manuscript through the review process. Thus, the corresponding author may need to expertly manage problems with the manuscript submission that may arise after a fellow, resident, or faculty member has taken another position.

A research project group meeting should include colleagues who are generating, collecting, or analyzing data, because these people may be included as authors on the final manuscript and are valuable sources of critical questions as the project moves along.

Collection, Assessment, and Analysis of Data

Getting started means choosing the right methods. I always check with the designated statistician before starting an educational research project to make sure that the methods are not going to be the Achilles heel, which will prevent me from publishing the data I have collected. In addition to your statistician, meet with your research team before you begin collecting data to visualize any glitches that could derail your project. Have your ultimate questions and goals in mind. Write a proposal in abstract form, to focus on your methods, imagined results, and desired endpoints. Are you measuring USMLE, Step 1 or Step 2, scores, final exam scores, faculty, resident, student satisfaction, observed skills in an OSCE or simulation laboratory? Give the proposed abstract of your tentative study to the statistician, who will determine if the methods being used will achieve the desired results. You may wish to have a group exposed to the intervention and compare it to a similar group without intervention, if you are able to do this educationally. You can also compare current data to historic controls to report whether outcomes are different with the new intervention compared to a historic preintervention control group of similar size and composition.

Funding of the Research Project

How much money will the study cost? Do you have funding? Is funding available for small research projects that are pilot projects? Your medical school may fund a small pilot project by giving you salary support for a short period to get your project up and running. Alternatively, funds may be available for statistical support, supplies, or travel for you to present your research study at a national or regional meeting. Apply for medical school small-fund grants; they are often easy to apply for and have a good chance of being funded (Carline 2004). Alternatively, some medical schools, such as the Mayo Medical School, have developed clinician-educator awards, to encourage innovation in medical education research (Viggiano, Shub, and Giere 2000).

Institutional Review Board

It is best to assume that it will be necessary to obtain approval from the Institutional Review Board (IRB) if you wish to study students' grades, aggregate scores, final exam scores, attitudes, course, faculty, tutor evaluations, or other methods of determining the utility of your intervention. Some medical schools have each student sign a consent form as he or she enters the school indicating that the school may use his or her anonymous responses to course evaluations and other questionnaires as research material. If students participate in focus groups, then individual consent forms are needed. If your medical school has not had students sign a consent form as they enter medical school, then you need to ask your medical school IRB whether you will be able to use student responses for research data without a specific informed consent form being signed. Even with universal student consent, you will still need IRB approval for your study. Your project may turn out to be an exempt study because you will be using only aggregate data. All data will be coded and deidentified by the statistician. This deidentification step eliminates any link between a student or faculty member and a certain response or grade.

The medical school IRB exists to protect students and faculty privacy and safety as well as to help research get done in medical education (Carline et al. 2007). I have found the IRB administrators at Harvard Medical School to be wonderful sources of information, particularly if you talk with them from the beginning, as you are thinking through a project. The Harvard Medical School Web site notes that the mission of the Committee on Human Studies (CHS) is to "insure that all participants are protected from any unnecessary risk while involved in a research project, that they make an informed decision to participate, and whenever possible, that there is a benefit to the participant or to society from the research" (www.hms.harvard.edu/orsp/human). The other goal of CHS is to help investigators develop appropriate research protocols in accordance with government and university policies and within accepted ethical guidelines.

Become certified in human studies research as soon as possible because without the certification, your protocol cannot move ahead. Find out if your hospital certification will suffice. The certification process may take up to six hours; you need to complete a series of Web-based instruction sessions and multiple-choice exams. Once you recognize that your study may require IRB approval, contact your IRB group for advice. I recommend that, as soon as you have an outline of your study and the key personnel, you call or meet with your designated IRB administrator and ask questions about new project forms, time line for approval, informed consent forms, and the necessary online tests you and your co-investigators must take to show understanding of general human subjects protection and the specific rules of your school. A good question to ask is whether your hospital approval to do research based on IRB tests will be sufficient for your medical school IRB. Will you need to take two separate sets of exams to become certified in human subjects training? Another issue is whether the approval for your study will come from your hospital or needs to come from both the hospital and the medical school because it involves medical students during clinical rotations at a specific hospital. All these questions need to be raised, tackled, and then settled early through in-depth conversations among you as the researcher, your co-investigators, and the IRB administrator assigned to your project.

The IRB administrator will recognize roadblocks that need to be removed to obtain study approval. Frequently, this person will recommend another person to talk with before the study is submitted to the IRB. It is useful to understand the details of the path the proposal must take to be approved by the IRB, including what signatures are needed and from whom. Find out if the people whose signatures you need will be in town when you finish writing your IRB protocol. If not, rush to finish the protocol to obtain the necessary signatures so that your project can proceed. Be careful to understand who exactly the signers will be. Frequently, the title of the person who is to sign does not resemble any title you are familiar with. Ask specifically who this person is and why he or she is to sign. Recently, I had to spend several hours getting different people to sign an IRB proposal that was rejected by the front desk IRB administrator because of incorrect signatures. I had not asked the right questions about who was my designated "head of program" and who was the official "statistician" designate for a proposal going through another hospital's IRB. I had made assumptions that turned out to be wrong. Eventually, all was remedied, but the time investment and awkwardness of the situation linger in my mind. Had I done the proper homework and asked the IRB officials in this other institution who the titles referred to instead of guessing, I would have saved myself a lot of unnecessary work and embarrassment.

Remember to include in your IRB proposal any data that you may already have or any curriculum materials. Table 14.1 lists the sections that are standard for the IRB proposal at Harvard Medical School.

Informed Consent, Personnel Roster, Cover Letter, and Amendments

Informed consent forms need to follow strict guidelines. You may be required to write a script that you will use to recruit subjects and submit to the IRB for approval, along with the informed consent form for recruiting volunteers for focus groups or having faculty or student groups fill out questionnaires. If the study is approved, you will need to use this script verbatim for your recruitment efforts that require informed consent.

Remember that all the researchers who are on the roster may need to have exam certification and a curriculum vitae on file as a researcher with the IRB.

Table 14.1.   Standard Sections for the IRB Proposal at Harvard Medical School

Title
Principal investigator and contact information
Study personnel
Additional institutional review boards reviewing this study
Hypothesis and goals
Study procedures and methodologies
Participant selection
Statistical design
Randomization to control or intervention groups
Plan for confidentiality of data
Plan for monitoring of data for the safety of participants
Use of study results
Expected duration of the study
Funding, if applicable
Study site(s)
Research participant information
Data source information
Informed consent, if applicable
Investigator conflicts of interest

Source: Adapted from Committee on Human Studies Application, Harvard Medical School / Harvard School of Dental Medicine, Boston, Massachusetts.

The principal investigator and the statistician who will handle the data analysis are essential to have on the personnel roster.

The cover letter is an excellent place to succinctly state the goal of your study and whether you are asking for an expedited review, given that you will be analyzing data only in the aggregate and no informed consent is needed, or a full-board review, given the need for signed informed consent.

If some part of your study design changes or the need for informed consent is recognized after the protocol has been approved, then an amendment is generally required to proceed with the changes. Contact the IRB administrators. They will outline the essential steps and give you the time line of the next Board of Review, so you can prepare your amendment protocol in time.

Collecting and Interpreting Data

The data you collect are the foundation for the results section of your manuscript. These data may be course evaluations, student or faculty questionnaires, test scores, observational data on faculty or student attitudes, or other measures, such as performance scores in the OSCE, National Board exams, or residency examinations. Be sure to collect the data as carefully and completely as possible. Send encouraging e-mail or oral messages to students and faculty requesting them to fill out anonymous questionnaires. In a current project I am doing, students have been given several extra weeks to fill out course evaluations in order to improve the overall response rate.

Statistical analyses and the statistician's interpretation of these data will supply the meat of your results in a quantitative study. Are the results significant? Is the significance due to your new method or something else? Are the results close to significance? What future change might make them significant? What if no significance is found? What are the possible explanations for this? Do the results make sense in light of what is known already? Do they break new ground? What do they add to the current literature? What is different, innovative, or novel about the results and the methods you used? Is your method adaptable to other medical schools, courses, and clerkships? How and why can others use it?

Submitting Your Work to a Medical Education Journal

Some major print journals in the field of medical education are listed below in alphabetical order, with their Web site address for submission of an article:

- *Academic Medicine* (www.editorialmanager.com/acadmed)
- *Advances in Health Sciences Education* (www.editorialmanager.com/ahse/)
- *Medical Education* (med@mededuc.com)
- *Medical Teacher* (MedicalTeacher@dundee.ac.uk)
- *Teaching and Learning in Medicine* (http://mc.manuscriptcentral.com/htlm)

Other general medicine journals that publish high-quality educational articles and their Web sites are:

- *Annals of Internal Medicine* (https://acponline.org/authors)
- *Journal of the American Medical Association* (http://manuscripts.jama.com)
- *Journal of General Internal Medicine* (https://jgim.iusm.iu.edu)
- *New England Journal of Medicine* (http://authors.nejm.org)

Look at specialty journals to see if they accept educational strategy or technology articles. Ask the medical school librarian to help you in your efforts to find the right journal for your manuscript. Direct your attention to other, lesser-known medical education journals and consider online journals.

Because journals differ in what each requires for word limits, abstract length, and number of tables and figures, decide before you begin writing which journal you prefer to submit the manuscript to (Bligh and Brice 2005). Then go to the journal Web site to study it. Read recent issues. Is this journal the best place for your work? Does it publish articles with similar themes or questions? Will your article appear like a duck out of water or will it be swimming among friends? Avoid having to do a considerable amount of rewriting before submitting your work by heeding the journal's stated purpose, philosophy, and specific requirements.

A factor in getting your work accepted at some journals is your ability to follow the directions on the journal's Web site for the mechanics of submission. Read, reread, and read out loud the fine print that the journal has carefully laid out for submission of an article. To reiterate, each journal differs. Carefully note the number of words allowed for the abstract, the need for keywords and where to place them, where the affiliations and degrees of the authors are placed (some journals do not publish the degrees of the authors, but do require them in your online submission), the ability to acknowledge people who contributed in some way but are not authors. Do the people who are acknowledged need to sign an agreement to be acknowledged? Do you need to note in your cover letter that each acknowledged person agrees to be acknowledged? How do you list funding from private or public sources? When and how do you note that the material has been partially presented at a national meeting? What style are the references to be in? The reference format may require that all authors of an article, even if more than ten in number, be listed. More commonly, only the first three authors, followed by "et al.," are required. Do not guess at the style and format the journal expects. There is no guesswork in being accepted by a prestigious journal; there is pure work.

Once you have digested the facts at the journal's Web site and committed them to memory or outlined them, begin writing your article.

Abstract: Look for the journal's word count for an abstract. Stick to it exactly. In fact, be under by a few words. I recently had an education paper sent back for minor revisions partly because the abstract word count was too high, even though I was confident from a computer-generated word count that I was exactly at the desired word limit. Write the abstract when every part of the manuscript is at least a rough draft. The abstract serves as a method of advertising your bottom-line innovations, your significant results, and your logical conclusions. The final publishable abstract should be created after, not before, the paper.

Introduction and Discussion: Both the introduction and the discussion parts of your paper require knowledge and review of the pertinent background literature. Where does your innovation fit in? What came before? What was needed? Why did you pursue the line of inquiry you did? What led to your technique? Summarize both classic and current articles. The most important part of the paper ultimately is your discussion of how the data you have obtained on a new method or innovation make a significant and new contribution to the field of medical education.

Tables and Figures: Journals differ in the format requested for figures and tables. Follow the recommendations to the letter. Use a media expert at your hospital or school to create figures and tables if you or one of your team is not adept at these skills. Put figures in a format that will be accepted by the journal, whether it is tiff (.tif), jpeg (.jpg), or other type of file.

References: References should be in the proper format for the journal to which you are submitting. Read the authors' instructions several times and keep a copy close by as you type the paper. Some authors use a software program to help them verify, organize, and insert references. Are the references to be in brackets at the end of the sentence? Are they to be placed before or after the sentence period? Are the references to be indicated by superscript numbers? Are the references to be in parentheses within the text or at the end of the sentence? Are they to be alphabetized in the reference list or to appear in the order in which that they appear in the text? Answer all these questions at the beginning and save time later. Remember that one of the problems you face with a journal rejection is reorganizing the references according to the next journal's style before submitting it anew.

A cover letter to the editor of the journal indicating which associate editor may be best to review your paper is frequently required. Even if not required, you may wish to suggest which associate editor is preferable. Review the associate editor's recent publications and editorials to figure this out. In addition, many journals ask for names of potential reviewers. Give a lot of thought to whom you suggest. Avoid competitors who may view your work negatively, with or without being aware of their own bias against you. At several journals, you are able to list people who should not review your work. Talk with your team; they may have excellent suggestions for fair and expert reviewers.

Conflict of Interest Forms and Copyright Transfer / Copyright Assignment Forms: Begin worrying about the conflict of interest and copyright forms from the beginning of your submission. Although ultimately simple to fill out, these forms are often difficult to get back from your busy authors in a wide variety of locations. Occasionally an author, upon reading the copyright transfer or assignment form, which stipulates that an author must have contributed to the design and intellectual content of the study, generated, collected, and approved all analyses of the data, and carefully reviewed the revised and final manuscripts, will decide that he or she is not fully qualified. This tentative author will then be dropped as an author.

Allow sufficient time for these forms to be completed so that even the busiest author can complete the forms and fax or e-mail them back to you or your administrator. My administrator keeps a log of each author's name, type of form (conflict of interest or copyright transfer or assignment), whether he or she has sent one or both of them back, and the date the forms were received. With a running tally, it is easy to remind only those authors who are late in sending in the forms. While some journals request these forms at the start of the submission and review process, others ask for them at the time of the final submission, after all revisions have been made and the article has achieved a final acceptance. Check the journal Web site to be certain. If you have questions, call or e-mail the editorial office.

Categories of Acceptance and Rejection

When you receive your journal review, the ideal is to have your manuscript accepted with no revisions or with minor revisions; the next-best category is having the manuscript accepted, but with major revisions (Pugsley 2009). Less good is being given the chance to resubmit the article with major revisions, but with no guarantee of acceptance. Finally, an article may be rejected outright with no chance for resubmission. The journal is generally clear about which category your manuscript has been assigned to. However, if you have questions, call or e-mail the editor who handled your manuscript.

If your article is rejected outright, with no chance for resubmission, change the article in accord with the criticisms leveled at it by the rejecting journal. Even though this journal rejected it, the questions and corrections may be helpful in improving your manuscript. Following their suggestions will increase the chances that your paper will eventually be accepted. Never give up on getting your work published if you think you have a valid study. Rather, think creatively about which journals may view it positively, and send the manuscript to these journals. Be sure to check the requirements of the new journal for references, figures, tables, and word count (Pugsley 2009). Each journal has its own standards. You must conform to them to get published. There is a journal for every reasonable article. Find it.

Reprints

Now that many journal articles can be printed off the Internet in a PDF format, reprints are not as popular and are expensive. Balance the advantage of having glossy articles with color pictures, which you can send out or give out to your co-authors, supporters, family, and friends, against the expense of the reprint charges for your individual budget. Remember that the reprints must be ordered at the time your article is accepted, which may be six months before it is published. Usually, you cannot place the order for reprints after the paper has been published, so consider carefully how many reprints you want. When you are going up for promotion to full professor, promotion committees may ask for reprints of your articles, especially if you are publishing in the fields of pathology, radiology, gastrointestinal endoscopy, or dermatology, where high-quality color photographs and photomicrographs are frequently necessary to demonstrate the crucial findings. In these fields, it may well be worth the initial expense to have available reprints of your important articles with the full-color glossy figures. Alternatively, a good color printer may make reprints unnecessary. Remember to save ten to twenty-five reprints or color copies of each article for future promotion committees.

Submitting Meeting Abstracts: The Pros and Cons

Meeting abstracts are useful for organizing data, jelling thoughts concerning the significance of the data, learning the pertinent literature, gaining experience in presenting, improving the quality of the final manuscript, and obtaining future collaborators. I find poster presentations to be an excellent way to obtain criticisms and kudos before submitting a research paper to a journal. A good poster session is really one long question-and-answer session that permits you to learn what questions to ask next or which areas of data may need to be better explored. Oral presentations also generate relevant questions about methods and are excellent opportunities to receive suggestions for further educational experiments or data analyses before submitting to a journal. However, abstracts are also time-consuming to write clearly and concisely.

Although it is not expensive to submit the abstract, it is usually expensive to present at meetings. In addition, abstracts may not be permitted to be part of your curriculum vitae bibliography section, depending on your medical school's regulations. Thus, no bibliographic notation of your oral or poster presentation will appear, even though you were delighted that your abstract was selected for a major meeting, you did a great job of presenting, and you met many well-known people in your field who may turn out to be terrific mentors.

If you decide to submit an abstract, abstracts (250 words) of your partly completed or fully completed, but not yet published, research can be submitted each February to the major national meeting for medical education, the Association of American Medical Colleges' Research in Medical Education (RIME) section, for either a poster presentation or a ten-minute oral presentation (followed by five minutes of questions) at the Association of American Medical Colleges' (AAMC) annual meeting each November. Abstracts should report completed investigations that contribute to medical education research and practice. Abstracts can also discuss the results of smaller-scale pilot projects, exploratory studies, or segments of larger projects. Accepted abstracts will be posted online on the RIME annual meeting program Web site. Abstracts are presented as either a ten-minute oral presentation or a poster. The RIME Planning Committee will decide the format after the abstract has been accepted. The AAMC Web site (www.aamc.org) notes that acceptance of an abstract and its presentation does not interfere with the submission of the study as a research paper to subsequent RIME meetings or as a journal article for *Academic Medicine* or other medical education journal.

Abstracts can also be submitted to regional educational offshoots of the AAMC's Group on Educational Affairs (GEA). GEA welcomes people with professional responsibility for medical student, resident, and continuing medical education who are designated by deans, hospital directors, or academic societies. The GEA comprises four sections: research in medical education (RIME, undergraduate medical education (UME), graduate medical education (GME), and continuing medical education (CME). The annual GEA national meeting occurs each fall as part of the AAMC annual meeting, as does the RIME Conference, where abstracts and oral presentations of the latest in educational research are presented. The Innovations in Medical Education Exhibits (IME) are also shown at the annual AAMC meeting. Each of the four separate regional geographic groups of GEA—the Central Group (CGEA), Northeast Group (NE-GEA), Southern Group (SGEA), and Western Group (WGEA)—hosts an annual spring meeting. Abstracts are submitted to these spring meetings months in advance. These regional meetings are excellent places to get started in medical education by presenting your latest data to an enthusiastic and committed audience of geographically close potential collaborators. The regional meetings are also places to learn more about medical education in a smaller setting, which is conducive to observing exchanges among educators regarding techniques and methods for success.

Web-based Publication of Innovations in Medical Education

MedEdPortal is a peer-reviewed, free Web-based tool that increases collaboration across disciplines and institutions by permitting the exchange of educational materials, including slide presentations, assessment tools, virtual patient cases, and faculty development materials. The MedEdPortal 2.0 repository and Web site can be found at www.aamc.org/mededportal. The MedEdPortal site has a content and digital asset management system to place published resources online. All copyright and patient privacy issues are discussed at the time of submission to allow users around the world to download the published resources for educational purposes without legal infringement. Some 1,300 educational publications are available to download. According to Reynolds and Candler (2008), MedEdPortal's rapid growth indicates that it is meeting a significant need for medical educators. A search engine helps locate the educational material for others to use in improving their teaching skills. Authors can track usage of their innovations for promotion packets in a similar manner to the citation index, which is used to track basic science and clinical research articles. Consider this site for the dissemination of materials you have created that are not protected by copyright infringement clauses and contracts. Contact the editors and managers of the site through www.aamc.org/mededportal to discuss whether your material is suitable.

Invited Articles

Does the word *invited* review article change what you do? If a journal invites you to submit a review or an opinion piece, or you ask the journal if it is interested in your idea for an article, and the answer is yes, it is usually assumed that what you write will be accepted. But if your article undergoes peer review, you must answer the reviewer criticisms and change the article accordingly, or it will not be accepted by the journal, even though it was an invited review.

✂ TEACHING TIPS

1. Consider each educational innovation to be worthy of study.
2. Ask the right questions and generate hypotheses with the help of an interested research team.
3. Include a statistician from the start of the project to avoid costly errors in design.
4. Consult the medical school and hospital IRB as soon as the study design is crystallized to avoid subsequent delays.
5. MedEdPortal offers an online peer-reviewed Web site for educational innovations.
6. Focus on writing and publishing the paper rather than lavishing time and money on an abstract presentation.

✂ TAKE-HOME POINTS

- To gain recognition and promotion, you must publish; therefore, make everything you do a potential publication.
- Be open about authorship and expectations for all authors; it will save misunderstandings and wounded feelings later.
- Recognize that the order of authors and the number of authors will change over time; be flexible and fair.
- Follow all directions for submission on a journal's Web site, however tedious and time-consuming they may be.
- Involve professionals in the media department of your hospital or medical school to improve the quality of your tables, figures, and drawings.
- If your study is rejected, find out why; fix the problem and submit to a different journal.

CHAPTER FIFTEEN

Promotion

- What are promotion boards looking for?
- How do I move up the ladder for promotion?
- When should I make an appointment to meet with a senior faculty member, department chair, or dean to determine if I am eligible for promotion?
- How do I identify the right recommenders for my promotion?
- Is there a best way to ask someone to write a letter for my promotion?

Promotion Tracks and Their Requirements for Teaching

Promotion on any of the three tracks—investigator, clinical, or teaching—usually depends on ample evidence of very good to excellent teaching evaluations. I frequently meet medical school faculty members in my department for the first time when they are going up for promotion. The chair of the department or a dean recognizes that they are without a teaching credential and sends them to me or another course director. These faculty members actively seek to be quickly involved in teaching and are highly motivated to do well. They almost always obtain the very good to excellent evaluations they need to bolster their claim of being the classic triple threat in academic medicine.

Clinical expertise, coupled with research and teaching excellence, is an impressive package to present for promotion. But is promotion, as important as it is, the only reason to be better? Remember the great teachers, who made the drudgery and endless sleeplessness of medical school, residency, and fellowship seem worthwhile? Wouldn't it be fun, satisfying, and rewarding to be in their honored league? What was it that they did to energize us? What was it that made us go back to our rooms, wards, or clinics with a sense of purpose, excitement, and renewed commitment? If promotion is not a priority for your career, remember how important excellent teaching is to learners. It is unforgettable.

Promotion on the Teacher-Clinician Track

If promotion is high on your priority list, being an award-winning teacher should help at the assistant professor level, but it is no guarantee, especially at the upper levels. Because there is a subjective element to awarding prizes in teaching, if promotion is to result, awards and prizes must be accompanied by other strengths, such as research and publication of educational studies, curriculum initiatives, model faculty development programs, or a national or an international presence, which is achieved by directing continuing medical education courses or receiving invitations to give keynote speeches at international symposia (Lovejoy and Clark 1995). Specifically, publication of teaching methods, writing about teaching styles, writing about results, and lecturing on teaching, writing chapters, and writing integrative reviews are all necessary at most medical schools to support the idea of scholarly efforts, as awards for excellent lecturing, small-group leadership, or graduate medical education activity are not. Rarely will a medical teacher be promoted above the level of associate professor with multiple teaching awards and no objective evidence of scholarship in medical education or national recognition due to educational offerings or courses. Full professor rank requires national and international recognition, something that is difficult to achieve in medical education. Levinson and Rubenstein (1999) recommended that the requirements for national and international recognition and for publication in peer reviewed journals on the clinician-teacher track be eliminated in favor of developing other, preferable methods of deciding excellence in the clinical and teaching realms. However, most medical schools continue to require publications and broad recognition for promotion. Fleming et al. (2005) recommended creating new yardsticks for clinician-educators that would be appropriate for their contributions to the academic medical center. Categories to consider documenting include teaching, mentoring and supervision, educational administration or service, and the scholarship of teaching.

Promotion to the top rank requires publication of research studies, textbooks, or position papers and invitations to be a visiting professor by other universities, medical schools, or educational organizations. Promotion to full professor comes with the recognition that you are sought after as a medical educator, innovator, faculty developer, or organizer of educational conferences or graduate medical education courses at a national or international level. You have made a significant and recognizable impact on your field. This recognition may include grants for educational research projects.

Trying to be promoted on the teacher-clinician track at most university medical schools is like climbing to the top of Mount Everest. A faculty survey at Johns Hopkins by Thomas et al. (2004) demonstrated that clinican-educator faculty were less likely to be at the higher ranks compared to faculty on the research tracks. A few people eventually manage to get to the top, but many people fail in various stages of their attempts. Those who fail may have fun in the process of trying, though those who do succeed in being promoted to full professor frequently need to try hard for a long time before they succeed.

Volunteer, nontenured faculty are important to the teaching mission of the Northeastern Ohio Universities College of Medicine. These faculty members were rewarded with a specific nontenure track, which recognizes productivity and excellence in teaching and standardizes the requirements for promotion (Williamson, Schrop, and Costa 2008). Northeastern Ohio Universities College of Medicine devised a system that recognizes scholarship in a broader manner than previously, with presentations at other institutions and at professional meetings being considered contributions equal to doing research.

Criteria for Promotion

Know where to find the latest set of criteria for promotion on the teacher-clinician track at your medical school. Review them carefully and then commit them to memory. They are the "must accomplish" immutable list. If you are going up on the teacher-clinician track, this means that your major area of excellence is in teaching or the clinical realm. A primary focus of excellence in teaching and educational leadership may be supported with activities in the clinical realm, laboratory or clinical investigation, education of patients, or service to the community, as well as administrative and institutional service. If your major focus has been clinical excellence, your minor area of supporting excellence may be in teaching or in basic research.

Spend as much time as necessary creating a curriculum vitae (CV) in the proper format, according to your medical school's promotion Web site. Generally, the font size is 12 for the body of the CV and size 14 for the titles of sections. Do not deviate from the requirements. The CV is essential to determining whether an individual clinician is ready for promotion. Hire a professional if you are not certain how to do the formatting or do not understand what the criteria mean or which category is the correct one for some of your contributions. Often someone at a hospital or medical school who is familiar with formatting CVs as part of his or her job is willing to moonlight. Otherwise, find a resume expert in your telephone Yellow Pages.

The CV at Harvard Medical School includes the following relevant areas for promotion on the teacher-clinician track:

1. Awards and honors, including all teaching award certificates and prizes, the year in which each was won, and what each award is for. List all nominations for teaching awards under a separate heading: "Teaching Award Nominations." Give the year for each, from the earliest to the most recent.

2. Narrative report of teaching, including innovations in curriculum creation, faculty development, clerkships, the design of nonprint materials, and Web site contributions, from the earliest to the most recent.

3. Report of teaching, including the following categories: local contributions to medical school courses and graduate medical courses, invited teaching presentations, visiting professorships and invited lectureships, symposium plenary lectures, and workshops at the local, national, and international level, from the earliest to the most recent.

4. Bibliography: This section of your CV should show each publication, curriculum offering, or Web-based case, with your name in bold in the author list, from the earliest to the most recent. This permits the promotions committee to quickly calculate the percentage of articles in which you are the first author, last (senior) author, or second author. The bibliography will have subsections, with the first usually being original articles. Promotion committees consider the original article section the most important part of your bibliography because the original articles represent your innovations in medical education, clinical research, and basic research.

In addition to creating your CV, pick your top ten papers. How do you do this? Look for papers in which you are the first, second, or last (senior) author. If you are second author, was this because you were mentoring the first author, who was a student, fellow, or resident? If you are last author, how did you contribute to the design, critical review of data, and methods, and did you help to write the manuscript? Are you in the senior author position as a mark of respect for an initial idea or input or because your laboratory facilities were used, but you had little other involvement with the day-to-day progress of the project and the writing of the manuscript? Be prepared to defend your position on a paper unless you were first author, in which case you are expected to have been the driving force behind the project since its inception and to have contributed substantially to the research methods, analysis of results, and writing of the discussion and conclusions.

The top ten papers should represent your best efforts in medical education, clinical research, and basic research. Even if you have not done basic research for twenty years, your papers from the time when you did do basic or clinical research are important to review for their impact on the field. Do your papers describe for the first time important innovations, a pathological process, technique, new therapy, epidemiological connection, or decisive clinical trial? One way to determine your impact on the field you published in is to see how many times your paper has been cited by subsequent authors. To do this for all of your original papers, go to the science citation index on the digital library Web site for your institution. Search all databases for your name, without your middle initial at first. Do this to cast the widest net for all your original papers. The ISI Web of Knowledge will indicate how many times each of your articles has been cited by other authors in their papers or reviews. It will also indicate the citations, giving the author, name of the paper, journal, year, volume, and pages. Put your middle initial in to search for additional original articles and reviews. The citation index permits you to see if your paper was cited only in the few years after it was published and then not at all, or has been cited recently by several authors. Determine which of your papers have been cited the most. Pick several of these to be in your top ten articles, especially if an article has been cited more than fifty times. To help finalize your choices, put your original articles in separate piles for teaching/education, clinical/epidemiological reports, clinical research, and basic research. If you are on the teacher-clinician ladder, put your best integrative review articles into a separate pile. Ask the chairperson who is proposing you to help you finalize your top ten. Bring along reprints of your original articles and the best review articles for your chairperson to consider. Even though review articles are not original articles, they may have a significant impact on doctors' understanding of an area, especially if you clarify and distill a field well. As a teacher, you are expected to be outstanding at clarifying and streamlining complex concepts. An excellent review article will show your prowess.

Reprints are expensive. You saved the high-quality reprints for a reason, and promotion is that reason. Many researchers do not routinely order reprints because the PDF of their article will be available online to send to those who want it. However, reprints or good color copies are particularly important in fields in which it is crucial to see images in full color or rich detail, such as pathology, gastrointestinal endoscopy, electron microscopy, immunocytochemistry, cytology, radiology, and dermatology. If you order reprints, *never* give away all of them. Rather, photocopy the paper for those who want it when you are down to your last ten to twenty-five reprints. Label and save in a safe, dry area these ten to twenty-five reprints for future promotion committees, even if the possibility of promotion seems long in the future. Search your hospital office or home office to find reprints of your original and review articles. If you find none, spend the money to have the original article from the medical library's collection photocopied on top-quality paper with a slight gloss. Promotion committees will ask for articles as reprints because the higher-quality paper makes visual images, tables, and figures easier to analyze and appreciate.

Once you have picked your top ten articles, put them in chronological order. You may wish to have them in chronological groupings by area of expertise, such as teaching, clinical innovation, basic research, and clinical research. After listing the citation, in which you **bold** your name, give a brief explanation (two to four sentences) of why each article or review is important to the field, moved the field along, was the first to describe, brought about changes in diagnosis or treatment, etc. Most members of your initial committee will have little detailed knowledge of the field you are an expert in; help them understand the importance of your work in a simple, straightforward, but positive and upbeat manner that capitalizes on the lasting significance of your work. The annotated top ten list is also the place to indicate your relationship to the first author, if you are not the first author on the paper (e.g., "the first author [give name] was a first-year medical student in my laboratory who designed and carried out research experiments with my guidance" or "the first author [give name] was a second-year fellow in my laboratory"). This clarification of who the first author was and what rank he or she held while in your laboratory solidifies your reputation for being a good mentor and a generous investigator, who is willing to give the trainee or student first authorship if he or she wrote the paper under your guidance.

In addition to original articles, the bibliography should include chapters, reviews, textbooks, and syllabi. Indicate by **bolding** your name in the author lineup. In addition, organize curricula, Web-based training modules or courses, technologies such as simulation, policy statements, and assessment tools by year. Give author(s) and the complete title for each as well as noting funding source(s), the amount of funding, and sponsoring organization.

Curriculum Vitae Formats at Different Medical Schools

I noted minor differences in the required curriculum vitae formats for promotion at Yale University Medical School, Johns Hopkins University Medical School, Weill Medical College of Cornell University, the University of Michigan Medical School, and the University of California, San Francisco Medical Center, compared to the Harvard Medical School format. Specifically, at Yale, honors and awards, lectures, and grants are cited from most recent to earliest, while publications are cited from earliest to most recent. At Johns Hopkins, appointments, grants, department administrative appointments and activities are listed from most recent to earliest, while publications and lectures are cited from earliest to most recent. At Weill Medical College, publications are listed from most recent to earliest. At the University of Michigan, the teaching section of the CV may be replaced by an educator's portfolio, references begin from earliest to most recent, and abstracts are included, beginning with the earliest and going to the most recent (www.umcranialbase.org/medschool/faculty/promopackage/AppendC_CVguidelines.PDF). The University of California, San Francisco, Medical Center uses earliest date to most recent date throughout its CV, and professional activities are divided into extramural and intramural listings.

Steps to Promotion

Once your CV is complete and correctly formatted and you have your top papers in order, schedule a meeting with the dean for faculty affairs or the designated faculty mentor interested in promotions at your medical school. If there is no such position, make an appointment with a professor at your school who can evaluate the quality of your CV and your teaching and clinical contributions. I recommend that this meeting take place long before scheduling a meeting with your division or department chair so that you are aware of the pluses and minuses of your application for promotion and can fix any deficiencies before you sit with your chair to discuss your possible promotion. The dean for faculty affairs is paid to get people promoted from all departments in an unbiased manner, whereas the chair has many mouths to feed. Never wait for the chair of your department or the divisional chief to say you are ready to be promoted. Be proactive and recommend yourself for promotion after careful review of the criteria and a meeting with a dean or knowledgeable professor who agrees that you have fulfilled each of the criteria fully and are ready for promotion. Other worthy candidates who have the chair's ear may be ahead of you on the promotion ladder for the same academic rank in your division or department, so it behooves you to look out for your own advancement.

Send your CV to the dean, professor, or department or division chair several days to a week before your meeting with him or her. If your CV is an accurate representation of what you have done and fulfills the criteria outlined by your medical school for promotion, the chair may say that you are a "slam dunk" for the rank you are going for. On the other hand, the chair or dean may point out areas in which you do not quite fulfill the criteria for leadership, international invitations, original articles, or funded research. The chair or dean's meeting will usually concentrate on the specific strengths and weaknesses of your portfolio package. Be prepared to succinctly discuss each clinical, research, administrative, and teaching activity. Know your CV completely, down to the last lecture and mentored resident or fellow. Awards and prizes will count more for assistant and associate ranks than for full professor rank. No awards you win may be enough to swing the promotion at any rank without evidence of research, mentoring, and publication in the area of medical teaching.

Letters of Recommendation

Recommendations for promotion are crucial, and you should give much thought to deciding whom to ask for a recommendation. When you have corrected any deficiencies in your promotion portfolio and CV, think about the faculty at your institution and around the country and the world who know your clinical ability, your research, and your teaching. Who has shared complex patients with you over the years? Who has been a collaborator or a chair of a committee that you contributed significantly to? Think about the faculty who have been consistently effusive in their praise of your abilities, teaching prowess, published work, lectures, grand rounds, or ability to run an educational course or initiative. Think of fellow national committee members you have worked with extensively and who have been loud in their approval of your work. Think back to the people who wrote letters for your last promotion; you impressed them once and may impress them again. Make a long list of possible recommenders, and then put the pros and cons next to each name in tabular format. Have they seen you teach? Have they reported their delight or approval of your work to you? Have they been a positive reviewer of a paper or a grant? Did they spontaneously volunteer in the past to write an excellent letter for promotion? Are they a competitor? Do they stand to gain or lose from your promotion? Do not take chances with an unknown quantity. Choose certain bets for recommendation-letter writers so that you can relax about the excellence and enthusiasm of the letters during the months to years when your promotion package makes its rounds. Recognize that if you are going up for full professor, your medical school may require that all letters come from full professors; no associate or assistant professor may be permitted to write in support of you. At some medical schools, certain letters must come from your peers who are doing the same type of work at other medical schools. It pays to start thinking about the possible letter writers well in advance. At national meetings during the months leading up to your proposal for promotion, take the opportunity to reintroduce yourself to former professors, research colleagues you may not have seen for a while, and former fellows who are now full professors. Gauge whether a particular person is cordial, is effusive, and cares enough about you to be a possible recommendation-letter writer.

Consult your chairperson, who is putting you up for promotion, regarding the possible letter writers. She or he often knows that a certain letter writer never writes effusive, warm, and positive letters but rather is always bent on backstabbing everyone just enough to derail the possible promotion. Contact potential recommendation-letter writers by phone or meet with them in person to determine the warmth of their tone and their exact words in response to your invitation to write a letter for your promotion. If it is, "Hooray!" "I can't wait for this to happen," or the classic, "Long overdue!" name this person as a recommendation-letter writer of the first order. You should be able to spot the great letter writer as the person who says your work is highly deserving, original, a major contribution, or a remarkable innovation in the field. If you hear tentativeness or lack of enthusiasm in the potential recommendation-letter writer's voice, or in an e-mail message, do not put this person on your final list.

If you are going up for promotion as an assistant or associate professor, your letter writers may be associate professors as well as full professors. Put professors on your list who express enthusiasm and say they are honored by your request. Having the recommendation of a giant in the field you are being promoted in is helpful, but it will not make up for a mediocre or lackluster letter. Be wary of peers who are going up for promotion to the same rank in the near future at your or another institution. They may not be the most objective judges of your merits as they try to achieve their own goals.

If you are meeting with the dean for faculty promotions, he or she will usually ask about support for the promotion from the department or divisional chair. Without such support, it may be difficult to achieve promotion. Try to gauge if the department chair is enthusiastic, even though your division chief may not be. The department chair may see something in your application that the divisional chief is unable to see. He or she may be able to persuade your division chief to support you. Although this backdoor maneuvering may work and get you promoted, it could create long-lived animosity between you and your divisional chief. At the full-professor level, you will need strong support from your department chair, divisional chair, hospital promotion committees, and medical school promotion committees before you become a realistic candidate for promotion.

At the full-professor level, your promotion pathway may be through two or more internal hospital promotion committees, which determine the strength of your packet before recommending that you go to the medical school for three or more committees. Some medical schools create a special committee for each candidate going up for the rank of full professor. This committee is charged with determining whether the quality of your work and its impact, and your leadership, innovations, and publications, are on a par with or better than full professors at comparable institutions. The path to full professor may take two to three years to complete, even if the medical school accepts your promotion packet as worthy of consideration.

Chair's Letter to the Promotion Committee

If your chair is not familiar with your work or your area of expertise, consider asking if you can help by writing your own first draft of the letter extolling your virtues and the reasons why you are ready for promotion to a certain rank. Although initially writing your own letter for promotion may seem odd, it makes sense when you consider that you know your innovations, expertise, and leadership activities better than anyone else. You might as well point them out in the most cogent way possible. The letter should summarize your major area of excellence and your achievements, contributions, and impact in this area. If your area is teaching, then you may have support for your promotion from your clinical expertise and innovation or basic or clinical investigation. The letter usually goes through multiple iterations, between your and your chair's revisions, before it goes into your promotion packet. Remember to focus on the achievements, leadership activities, and invitations from national and international sources that have occurred since your last promotion, whether that was to the assistant or associate professor level. Your top ten papers, however, may well be from your years as an instructor or assistant professor, when you were active as a researcher before you shifted into medical education. Among the top ten papers, only a few may be from the medical education literature, if you recently switched career goals from the clinical realm to the medical education track.

Failure to Be Promoted

Do not "test the waters" when you begin your climb up the promotion ladder toward a specific rank. Either you have met the listed immutable criteria or you have not. If you have met the criteria, move ahead with confidence and with your head held high. If, however, you are hoping for the best and for good will on the part of the promotion committee, forget being put up for promotion until you are truly ready. Failure to attain promotion usually means that you were put up too soon by your chair, with not enough evidence of academic scholarship in the form of grants, original articles, reviews, chapters, books, or national and international speaking invitations, all of which indicate that you are an acknowledged expert in your field. The committee on promotions may suggest that you try again after several more papers, books, reviews, have been published, more grants have been received, increased leadership experience has been demonstrated, and national or international invitations are in evidence. The time line to complete these requirements, including the publications and grants, and to achieve a noticeable impact in your field may be on the order of three to five years. If you are willing to generate the grant revenue and the publications, you will likely achieve promotion in the future, with expert guidance throughout the process from your chair or a dean.

The second most common reason for not being promoted at the upper levels is that the promotion is blocked by one or more professors who are unenthusiastic about the quality of your work, its impact, and its importance on the field. These professors do not think that you should join their ranks as an associate or a full professor. If you recognize that you have an enemy on one of the promotion committees, alert your chair or dean to this fact. It may prevent your being blocked by this person. When you submit an article to a journal, you are asked to alert the editors to reviewers who should not review your manuscript because of acknowledged past problems or animosity. Going up for promotion is similar in that you may wish to give a list to your chairperson of people who cannot evaluate you fairly. Some of these people could be on one of your promotion committees or be best friends with promotion committee members.

What if Promotion Is Denied?

If, despite your best efforts, your promotion is denied or blocked at your institution, consider moving to another institution after discussing your chances for promotion there. What is denied to you at one institution may be given to you in a flash at another. I have happy friends who are thriving professors at other institutions after being denied or blocked for promotion to full professor at their original institution.

✒ TAKE-HOME POINTS

- Begin years ahead to prepare for your desired promotion. Save at least ten reprints of original articles for your ultimate promotion packet; the eventual impact, in the fields in which visual images count, is worth the initial cost.
- Produce an accurate and complete CV for teaching contributions.
- Avoid going up for promotion until you have clearly fulfilled all the publication, innovation, and leadership criteria expected at the rank you are seeking; disappointment and disillusionment can be the result.
- Choose recommendation-letter writers at the correct rank who enthusiastically endorse you and your work. Ask for the recommendation letter by phone or in person to better judge the enthusiasm.
- Promotion criteria are inflexible; you must meet them.
- Deans are available for advice. Follow their advice.
- Write your own chairperson's letter for your promotion, describing how you have more than adequately fulfilled each of the rank's requirements; you are your own best salesperson.
- If your promotion process is not going well, find out why and try to fix the problem.
- If your promotion does not go through, get promoted at another medical school.

References

Aagaard, E., A. Teherani, and D. M. Irby. 2004. Effectiveness of the one-minute preceptor model for diagnosing the patient and the learner: Proof of concept. *Acad Med* 79:42–49.

AAMC/HHMI Committee Report. Alpern, R. J., and S. Long. 2009. *Scientific Foundations for Future Physicians*. www.hhmi.org/grants/sffp.html.

Alexander, E. K. 2008. Perspective: Moving students beyond an organ-based approach when teaching medical interviewing and physical examination skills. *Acad Med* 83:906–9.

Alguire, P. C. 1998. A review of journal clubs in postgraduate medical education. *J Gen Intern Med* 13:347–53.

Alguire, P. C., D. E. De Witt, L. E. Pinsky, and G. S. Ferenchick. 2008. *Teaching in Your Office: A Guide to Instructing Medical Students and Residents*. 2nd ed. Philadelphia: American College of Physicians.

Allen, D., and K. Tanner. 2005. Infusing active learning into the large-enrollment biology class: Seven strategies from the simple to complex. *Cell Biol Educ* 4:262–68.

Al-Mateen, C. S. 2008. Team-based learning in a psychiatry clerkship. In *Team-based Learning for Health Professions: A Guide to Using Small Groups for Improving Learning*, ed. L. K. Michaelsen, D. X. Parmelee, K. K. McMahon, and R. E. Levine, 195–201. Sterling, VA: Stylus Publishing.

Anderson, L. W., D. R. Krathwohl, and B. S. Bloom. 2001. *A Taxonomy for Learning, Teaching and Assessing: A Revision of Bloom's Taxonomy of Educational Objectives*. Abridged ed. New York: Addison Wesley Longman.

Andreatta, P. B., and L. D. Gruppen. 2009. Conceptualising and classifying validity evidence for simulation. *Med Educ* 43:1028–35.

Appavu, S. K. 2009. Two decades of simulation-based training: Have we made progress? *Crit Care Med* 37:2843–44.

Armstrong, E. G. 1991. A hybrid model of problem-based learning. In *The Challenge of Problem Based Learning*, ed. D. Boud and G. Feletti, 137–49. London: Kogan Page.

Armstrong, E. G., and C. M. Christensen. Harvard Macy Institute's Program: Leading Innovations in Health Care and Education. Apply to: Harvard_Macy@hms.harvard.edu.

Armstrong, E. G., J. Doyle, and N. L. Bennett. 2003. Transformative professional development of physicians as educators: Assessment of a model. *Acad Med* 78:702–8.

Barnes, L. B., C. R. Christensen, and A. J. Hansen. 1994a. Premises and practices of discussion teaching. In *Teaching and the Case Method*. 3rd ed., ed. L. B. Barnes, C. R. Christensen, and A. J. Hansen, 23–34. Boston: Harvard Business School Press.

Barnes, L. B., C. R. Christensen, and A. J. Hansen. 1994b. Teaching with cases at the

Harvard Business School. In *Teaching and the Case Method*. 3rd ed., ed. L. B. Barnes, C. R. Christensen, and A. J. Hansen, 34–68. Boston: Harvard Business School Press.

Barrows, H. S. 1988. *The Tutorial Process*. Springfield, IL: Southern Illinois University School of Medicine.

Barrows, H. S., and R. M. Tamblyn. 1980. *Problem-Based Learning: An Approach to Medical Education*. Vol. 1. New York: Springer Publishing Co.

Barsuk, J. H., W. C. McGahie, E. R. Cohen, K. J. O'Leary, and D. B. Wayne. 2009. Simulation-based mastery learning reduces complications during central venous catheter insertion in a medical intensive care unit. *Crit Care Med* 37:2697–2701.

Bass, E. B. 2009. Problem identification and general needs assessment. In *Curriculum Development for Medical Education*. 2nd ed., ed. D. E. Kern, P. A. Thomas, and M. T. Hughes, 10–26. Baltimore: Johns Hopkins University Press.

Beaumier, A., G. Bordage, D. Saucier, and J. Turgeon. 1992. Nature of the clinical difficulties of first-year family medicine residents under direct observation. *Can Med Assoc J* 146:489–97.

Beecher, A. C., J. C. Lindemann, J. A. Morzinski, and D. E. Simpson. 1997. Use of the educator's portfolio to stimulate reflective practice among medical educators: The educator's portfolio. *Teach Learn Med* 9:56–59.

Bennett, K. J., D. L. Sackett, R. B. Haynes, V. R. Neufeld, P. Tugwell, and R. Roberts. 1987. A controlled trial of teaching critical appraisal of the clinical literature to medical students. *JAMA* 257:2451–54.

Betancourt, J. R. 2003. Cross-cultural medical education: Conceptual approaches and frameworks for evaluation. *Acad Med* 78:560–69.

Bierer, S. B., E. F. Dannefer, C. Taylor, P. Hall, and A. L. Hull. 2008. Methods to assess students' acquisition, application and integration of basic science knowledge in an innovative competency-based curriculum. *Med Teach* 30:e171–77.

Bing-You, R. G., and R. L. Trowbridge. 2009. Why medical educators may be falling at feedback. *JAMA* 302:1330–31.

Bland, C. J., C. C. Schmitz, F. T. Stritter, J. A. Aluise, and R. C. Henry. 1990. *Successful Faculty in Academic Medicine: Essential Skills and How to Acquire Them*, 15–20. New York: Springer Publishing Co.

Bligh, J., and J. Brice. 2005. Research and publication. In *A Practical Guide for Medical Teachers*. 2nd ed., ed. J. A. Dent and R. M. Harden, 412–20. London: Elsevier / Churchill Livingstone.

Bloom, B. S., M. D. Engelhart, E. J. Furst, W. H. Hill, and D. R. Krathwohl. 1956. *Taxonomy of Educational Objectives. Handbook 1. Cognitive Domain*. New York: Longmans, Green and Co.

Bokken, L., T. Linssen, A. Scherpbier, C. van der Vleuten, and J. J. Rethans. 2009. Feedback by simulated patients in undergraduate medical education: A systematic review of the literature. *Med Educ* 43:202–10.

Bowen, J. 2005. Clinical teaching methods of the ambulatory setting. In *Guidebook for Clerkship Directors*. 3rd ed., ed. R.-M. E. Fincher, 109–15. Omaha, NE: Alliance for Clinical Education.

Brawer, J., Y. Steinert, J. St-Cyr, K. Watters, and S. Wood-Dauphinee. 2006. The significance and impact of a faculty teaching award: Disparate perceptions of department chairs and award recipients. *Med Teacher* 28:614–17.

Buchel, T. L., and F. D. Edwards. 2005. Characteristics of effective clinical teachers. *Fam Med* 37:30–35.

Bulpitt, C. J. 1987. Confidence intervals. *Lancet* 1:494–97.

Cain, J., and E. Robinson. 2008. A primer on audience-response systems: Current applications and future considerations. *Am J Pharm Educ* 72: article 77.

Caldwell, J. E. 2007. Clickers in the large classroom: current research and best-practice tips. *CBE Life Sci Educ* 6:9–20.

Cantillon, P. 2003. ABC of learning and teaching in medicine: Teaching large groups. *Br Med J* 326:437–40.

Carline, J. D. 2004. Funding medical education research: Opportunities and issues. *Acad Med* 79:918–24.

Carline, J. D., P. S. O'Sullivan, L. D. Gruppen, and K. Richardson-Nassif. 2007. Crafting successful relationships with the IRB. *Acad Med* 82:S57–60.

Chen, F. M., H. Bauchner, and H. Burstin. 2004. A call for outcomes research in medical education. *Acad Med* 79:955–60.

Christensen, C. R. 1991a. The discussion teacher in action: Questioning, listening and response. In *Education for Judgment: The Artistry of Discussion Leadership,* ed. C. R. Christensen, D. A. Garvin, and A. Sweet, 153–72. Boston: Harvard Business School Press.

Christensen, C. R. 1991b. Premises and practice of discussion teaching. In *Education for Judgment: The Artistry of Discussion Leadership,* ed. C. R. Christensen, D. A. Garvin, and A. Sweet, 15–34. Boston: Harvard Business School Press.

Cole, K. A., L. R. Barker, K. Kolodner, P. Williamson, S. M. Wright, and D. E. Kern. 2004. Faculty development in teaching skills: An intensive longitudinal model. *Acad Med* 79:469–80.

Collins, J. 2006. Education techniques for lifelong learning: Writing multiple-choice questions for continuing medical education activities and self-assessment modules. *RadioGraphics* 26:543 51.

Cook, D. A., G. Bordage, and H. G. Schmidt. 2008. Description, justification and clarification: A framework for classifying the purposes of research in medical education. *Med Educ* 42:128–33.

Cook, D. A., A. J. Levinson, S. Garside, D. M. Dupras, P. J. Erwin, and V. M. Montori. 2008. Internet-based learning in the health professions: A meta-analysis. *JAMA* 300:1181–96.

Covey, S. R. 1989. *The Seven Habits of Highly Effective People: Restoring the Character Ethic.* New York: Simon & Schuster.

Covey, S. R. 2004. *The Eighth Habit: From Effectiveness to Greatness.* New York: Simon & Schuster.

Cox, S. S., and M. S. Swanson. 2002. Identification of teaching excellence in operating room and clinic settings. *Am J Surg* 183:251–55.

Cruess, S. R., R. L. Cruess and Y. Steinert. 2008. Role modeling-making the most of a powerful teaching strategy. *BMJ* 336:718–21.

Crumlish, C. M., M. A. Yialamas, and G. T. McMahon. 2009. Quantification of bedside teaching by an academic hospitalist group. *J Hosp Med* 4:304–7.

Dannefer, E. F., and L. C. Henson. 2007. The Portfolio approach to competency-based assessment at the Cleveland Clinic Lerner College of Medicine. *Acad Med* 82:493–502.

Dauphinee, W. D., and S. Wood-Dauphinee. 2004. The need for evidence in medical education: The development of best evidence medical education as an opportunity to inform, guide, and sustain medical education research. *Acad Med* 79:925–30.

Davis, M. H., and R. M. Harden. 2003. Competency-based assessment: Making it a reality. *Med Teach* 25:565–68.

Davis, M. H., and G. G. Ponnamperuma. 2005a. Portfolios, projects and dissertations. In *A Practical Guide for Medical Teachers,* ed. J. A. Dent and R. M. Harden, 346–56. London: Elsevier/Churchill Livingston.

Davis, M. H., and G. G. Ponnamperuma. 2005b. Work-based assessment. In *A Practical Guide for Medical Teachers,* ed. J. A. Dent and R. M. Harden, 336–45. London: Elsevier/Churchill Livingston.

Deenadayalan, Y., K. Grimmer-Somers, M. Prior, and S. Kumar. 2008. How to run an effective journal club: A systematic review. *J Eval Clin Pract* 14:898–911.

Dent, J. A. 2005a. Ambulatory care teaching. In *A Practical Guide for Medical Teachers.* 2nd ed., ed. J. A. Dent and R. M. Harden, 86–95. London: Elsevier/Churchill Livingstone.

Dent, J. A. 2005b. Bedside teaching. In *A Practical Guide for Medical Teachers.* 2nd ed., ed. J. A. Dent and R. M. Harden, 77–85. London: Elsevier/Churchill Livingstone.

Dent, J. A., and E. A. Hesketh. 2003. Developing the teaching instinct. 9: How to teach in an ambulatory care (outpatient) teaching centre. *Med Teach* 25:488–91.

Diamond, R. M., L. F. Gardiner, and D. W. Wheeler. 2002. Requisites for sustainable institutional change. In *Field Guide to Academic Leadership,* ed. R. M. Diamond and B. E. Adam, 15–24. San Francisco: Jossey-Bass.

Dorfsman, M. L., and A. B. Wolfson. 2009. Direct observation of residents in the emergency department: A structured educational program. *Acad Emerg Med* 16:343–51.

Dunaway, G. A. 2005. Adaption of team learning to an introductory graduate pharmacology course. *Teach Learn Med* 17:56–62.

Edwards, K. S., P. K. Woolf, and T. Hetzler. 2002. Pediatric residents as learners and teachers of evidence-based medicine. *Acad Med* 77:748.

Elzubeir, M. A., and D. E. Rizk. 2001. Identifying characteristics that students, interns, and residents look for in their role models. *Med Educ* 35:272–77.

Ende, J. 1983. Feedback in clinical medical education. *JAMA* 250:777–81.

Ennis, R. H. 1962. A concept of critical thinking: A proposed basis for research in the teaching and evaluation of critical thinking ability. *Harvard Educ Rev* 32:81–111.

Ennis, R. H. 1985. A logical basis for measuring critical thinking skills. *Educ Leadership* 43 (2):44–48.

Evidence-Based Working Group. 1992. Evidence-based medicine: A new approach to teaching the practice of medicine. *JAMA* 268:2420–25.

Ferren, A. S., and W. W. Stanton. 2004. Leadership through Collaboration: The Role of the Chief Academic Officer. Westport, CT: Praeger.

Fincher, R.-E. 2005. Writing multiple-choice questions. In *Guidebook for Clerkship Directors.* 3rd ed., ed. R.-M. E. Fincher, 133–248. Omaha, NE: Alliance for Clinical Education.

Fitzgibbons, J. P., D. R. Bordley, L. R. Berkowitz, B. W. Miller, and M. C. Henderson. 2006. Redesigning residency education in internal medicine: A position paper from the Association of Program Directors in Internal Medicine. *Ann Intern Med* 144:920–26.

Fleming, V. M., N. Schnidler, G. J. Martin, and D. A. DaRosa. 2005. Separate and equitable promotion tracks for clinician-educators. *JAMA* 294:1101–4.

Friedman, B. D. M. 2005. Principles of assessment. In *A Practical Guide for Medical Teachers,* ed. J. A. Dent and R. M. Harden, 282–92. London: Elsevier/Churchill Livingstone.

Friedrich, M. J. 2002. Harvard Macy Institute helps physicians become better educators and change agents. *JAMA* 287:3197–99.

Galbraith, M. W. 1998. *Adult Learning Methods: A Guide for Effective Instruction.* 2nd ed. Malabar, FL: Krieger Publishing Co.

Garvin, D. A. 2003. Making the case: Professional education for the world of practice. *Harvard Magazine* 106:56–65.

Glicken, A. D., and G. B. Merenstein. 2007. Addressing the hidden curriculum: Understanding educator professionalism. *Med Teach* 29:54–57.

Godfrey, K. 1985. Simple linear regression in medical research. *N Engl J Med* 313:1629–36.

Greenwald, B. 1991. Teaching technical material. In *Education for Judgment: The Artistry of Discussion Leadership,* ed. C. R. Christensen, D. A. Garvin, and A. Sweet, 193–213. Boston: Harvard Business School Press.

Griffith, C. H., 3rd, J. F. Wilson, S. A. Haist, T. A. Albritton, B. A. Bognar, S. J. Cohen, C. J. Hoesley, M. J. Fagan, G. S. Ferenchick, O. W. Pryor, E. Friedman, H. E. Harrell, P. A. Hemmer, B. L. Houghton, R. Kovach, D. R. Lambert, T. H. Loftus, T. D. Painter, M. M. Udden, R. S. Watkins, and R. Y. Wong. 2009. Internal medicine clerkship characteristics associated with enhanced student examination performance. *Acad Med* 84:895–901.

Gronlund, N. E. 2006a. Writing selection items: Multiple choice. In *Assessment of Student Achievement.* 8th ed., 75–92. Boston: Pearson Education.

Gronlund, N. E. 2006b. Writing supply items: Short answer and essay. In *Assessment of Student Achievement.* 8th ed., 110–25. Boston: Pearson Education.

Gruppen, L. D. 2007. Improving medical education research. *Teach Learn Med* 19:331–35.

Gruppen, L. D., A. Z. Frohna, R. M. Anderson, and K. D. Lowe. 2003. Faculty development for educational leadership and scholarship. *Acad Med* 78:137–41.

Hafler, J. P. 1989. Case Writing at Harvard Medical School. EdD diss., Harvard Graduate School of Education, Harvard University.

Hafler, J. P., and F. H. Lovejoy Jr. 2000. Scholarly activities recorded in the portfolios of teacher-clinician faculty. *Acad Med* 75:649–52.

Haidet, P., K. J. O'Malley, and B. Richards. 2002. An initial experience with "team learning" in medical education. *Acad Med* 77:40–44.

Harden, R. M. 2002. Developments in outcome-based education. *Med Teach* 24:117–20.

Harden, R. M., and F. A. Gleeson. 1979. Assessment of clinical competence using an objective structured clinical examination (OSCE). *Med Educ* 13:41–54.

Harden, R. M., J. R. Crosby, and M. H. Davis. 1999. AMEE Guide No. 14. Outcome-based education. Part I: An introduction to outcome based education.

Hartzell, J. D., G. R. Veerappan, K. Posley, N. M. Shumway, and S. J. Durning. 2009. Resident run journal club: A model based on the adult learning theory. *Med Teacher* 31:e156–61.

Hatton, N. 1982. How to plan and deliver a lecture. In *The Medical Teacher*. 2nd ed., ed. K. R. Cox and C. E. Ewan, 29–36. New York: Churchill Livingstone.

Hebert, R. S., and S. M. Wright. 2003. Re-examining the value of medical grand rounds. *Acad Med* 78:1248–52.

Heneghan, C., and P. Glasziou. 2005. Evidence-based medicine. In *A Practical Guide for Medical Teachers*. 2nd ed., ed. J. A. Dent and R. M. Harden, 271–80. London: Elsevier / Churchill Livingstone.

Henzi, D., E. Davis, R. Jasinevicius, and W. Hendricson. 2007. In the students' own words: What are the strengths and weaknesses of the dental school curriculum? *J Dent Educ* 71:632–45.

Hesketh, E. A., G. Bagnall, E. G. Buckley, M. Friedman, E. Goodall, R. M. Harden, J. M. Laidlaw, L. Leighton-Beck, P. McKinlay, R. Newton, and R. Oughton. 2001. A framework for developing excellence as a clinical educator. *Med Educ* 35:555–64.

Hill, A. 2007. Continuous curriculum assessment and improvement: A case study. *New Directions for Teaching and Learning* 112:33–44.

Ho, M.-J., G. Yao, K.-L. Lee, M. C. Beach, and A. R. Green. 2008. Cross-cultural medical education: Can patient-centered cultural competency training be effective in non-Western countries? *Med Teach* 30:719–21.

Holmboe, E. S. 2004. Faculty and the observation of trainees' clinical skills: Problems and opportunities. *Acad Med* 79:16–22.

Holmboe, E. S., M. Yepes, F. Williams, and S. J. Huot. 2004. Feedback and the Mini-Clinical Evaluation Exercise. *J Gen Intern Med* 19:558–61.

Holst, R., C. J. Funk, H. S. Adams, M. Bandy, C. M. Boss, B. Hill, C. B. Joseph, and R. K. Lett. 2009. Vital pathways for hospital librarians: Present and future roles. *J Med Libr Assoc* 97:285–92.

Hurst, J. W. 1999. *Teaching Medicine: Process, Habits, and Actions*. Atlanta: Scholars Press.

Irby, D. M. 1992. How attending physicians make instructional decisions when conducting teaching rounds. *Acad Med* 67:630–38.

Irby, D. M., P. G. Ramsey, G. M. Gillmore, and D. Schaad. 1991. Characteristics of effective clinical teachers of ambulatory care medicine. *Acad Med* 66:54–55.

Issenberg, S. B., W. C. McGaghie, I. R. Hart, J. W. Meyer, J. M. Flener, E. R. Petrusa, R. A. Waugh, D. D. Brown, R. R. Safford, I. H. Gessner, D. L. Gordon, and G. A. Ewy. 1999. Simulation technology for health care professional skills training and assessment. *JAMA* 282:861–66.

Issenberg, S. B., W. C. McGaghie, E. R. Petrusa, D. L. Gordon, and R. J. Scalese. 2005. What are the features and uses of high-fidelity medical simulations that lead to most effective learning? BEME Guide no. 4. *Med Teach* 27:10–28.

Jenicek, M., and D. L. Hitchcock. 2005. *Evidence-Based Practice: Logic and Critical Thinking in Medicine*. Chicago: American Medical Association Press.

Jha, V., N. D. Quinton, H. L. Bekker, and T. E. Roberts. 2009. Strategies and interventions for the involvement of real patients in medical education: A systematic review. *Med Educ* 43:10–20.

Kaagan, S. S. 1997. *Leadership Lessons: From a Life of Character and Purpose in Public Affairs*. Lanham, MD: University Press of America.

Kasulis, T. P. 1984. Questioning. In *The Art and Craft of Teaching*, ed. M. M. Gullette, 39–48. Cambridge, MA: Harvard University Press.

Kelly, P. A., P. Haidet, V. Schneider, N. Searle, C. L. Seidel, and B. F. Richards. 2005. A comparison of in-class learner engagement across lecture, problem-based learning and team learning using the STROBE classroom observation tool. *Teach Learn Med* 17:112–18.

Kemp, J. E., G. R. Morrison, and S. M. Ross. 1994. Developing evaluation instruments. In *Designing Effective Instruction,* 180–213. New York: Macmillan College Publishing Co.

Kern, D. E., P. A. Thomas, and M. T. Hughes. 2009. *Curriculum Development for Medical Education: A Six-Step Approach.* 2nd ed. Baltimore: Johns Hopkins University Press.

Kitchen, E., J. D. Bell, S. Reeve, R. R. Sudweeks, and W. S. Bradshaw. 2003. Teaching cell biology in the large-enrollment classroom: Methods to promote analytical thinking and assessment of their effectiveness. *Cell Biol Educ* 2:180–94.

Knight, J. K., and W. B. Wood. 2005. Teaching more by lecturing less. *Cell Biol Educ* 4:298–310.

Knowles, M. S. 1990. *The Adult Learner: A Neglected Species.* 4th ed. Houston: Gulf Publishing Co.

Knowles, M. S., E. F. Holton III, and R. A. Swanson. 2005. *The Adult Learner: The Definitive Classic in Adult Education and Human Resource Development.* 6th ed. Amsterdam: Elsevier.

Koch, K. 1993. The stomach. In *Atlas of Gastrointestinal Motility in Health and Disease,* ed. M. M. Schuster, 163. Baltimore: Williams & Wilkins.

Kogan, J. R., E. S. Holmboe, and K. E. Hauer. 2009. Tools for direct observation and assessment of clinical skills of medical trainees: A systematic review. *JAMA* 302:1316–26.

Koh, G. C.-H., H. E. Khoo, M. L. Wong, and D. Koh. 2008. The effects of problem-based learning during medical school on physician competency: A systematic review. *CMAJ* 178:34–41.

Kohn, L. T., J. M. Corrigan, and M. S. Donalson, eds. 1999. *To Err Is Human: Building a Safer Health System.* Washington, DC: National Academy Press.

Kolb, D. A. 1984. *Experiential Learning: Experience as the Source of Learning and Development.* Englewood Cliffs, NJ: Prentice Hall.

Kumagai, A. K., and M. L. Lypson. 2009. Beyond cultural competence: Critical consciousness, social justice, and multicultural education. *Acad Med* 84:782–87.

Lawler, E. M., X. M. Chen, and E. A.Venso. 2007. Student perspectives on teaching techniques and outstanding teachers. *J Scholar Teach Learn* 7:32–48.

LeBlond, R. F., R. L. DeGowin, and D. D. Brown. 2004. The abdomen. In *DeGowin's Diagnostic Examination: The Complete Guide to Assessment, Examination, Differential Diagnosis.* 8th ed., 509–608. New York: McGraw-Hill.

Lee, G.-H., Y.-H. Lin, K.-I. Tsou, S.-J. Shiau, and C. S. Lin. 2009. When a problem-based learning tutor decides to intervene. *Acad Med* 84:1406–11.

Lesky, L. G., and W. Y. Hershman. 1995. Practical approaches to a major educational challenge: Training students in the ambulatory setting. *Arch Intern Med* 155:897–904.

Levinson, W., and A. Rubenstein. 1999. Mission critical: Integrating clinician-educators into academic medical centers. *N Engl J Med* 341:840–43.

Levinson, W., and A. Rubenstein. 2000. Integrating clinician-educators into academic medical centers: Challenges and potential solutions. *Acad Med* 75:906–12.

Levinson, W., D. L. Roter, J. P. Mullooly, V. T. Dull, and R. M. Frankel. 1997. Physician-patient communication: The relationship with malpractice claims among primary care physicians and surgeons. *JAMA* 277:553–59.

Linthorst, G. E., J. M. Daniels, and D. J. van Westerloo. 2007. The majority of bold statements expressed during grand rounds lack scientific merit. *Med Educ* 41:965–67.

Linzer, M., J. T. Brown, L. M. Frazier, E. R. DeLong, and W. C. Siegel. 1988. Impact of a medical journal club on house-staff reading habits, knowledge, and critical appraisal skills: A randomized control trial. *JAMA* 260:2537–41.

Lovejoy Jr., F. H., and M. B. Clark. 1995. A promotion ladder for teachers at Harvard Medical School: Experience and challenges. *Acad Med* 70:1079–86.

Lowenstein, R., G. Fernandez, and L. A. Crane. 2007. Medical school faculty discontent: prevalence and predictors of intent to leave academic careers. *BMC Med Educ* 7:37–44.

Ludmerer, K. M. 1999. *Time to Heal.* New York: Oxford University Press.

Manfred, L. 2005. Clinical teaching methods for the inpatient setting. In *Guidebook for Clerkship Directors.* 3rd ed., ed. R.-M. E. Fincher, 104–9. Omaha, NE: Alliance for Clinical Education.

Markert, R. J. 1989. A research methods and statistics journal club for residents. *Acad Med* 64:223–24.

Markert, R. J. 2001. What makes a good teacher? Lessons from teaching medical students. *Acad Med* 76:809–10.

Marks, M., and S. Humphrey-Murto. 2005. Performance assessment. In *A Practical Guide for Medical Teachers,* ed. J. A. Dent and R. M. Harden, 323–35. London: Elsevier/Churchill Livingston.

Marzano, R. J., and J. S. Kendall. 2007. *The New Taxonomy of Educational Objectives.* 2nd ed. Thousand Oaks, CA: Corwin Press.

Mayer, D. 2004. *Essential Evidence-Based Medicine.* Cambridge: Cambridge University Press.

McAleer, S., and E. A. Hesketh. 2003. Developing the teaching instinct. 10: Assessment. *Med Teach* 25:585–88.

McArdle, P. J. 2007. Innovations in undergraduate medical education and in graduate medical training. *J Cont Educ Health Prof* 17:214–23.

McDonald, F. S., S. L. Zeger, and J. C. Kolars. 2008. Associations of conference attendance with internal medicine in-training examination scores. *Mayo Clin Proc* 83:449–53.

McGaghie, W. C. 1999. Simulation in professional competence assessment: Basic considerations. In *Innovative Simulations for Assessing Professional Competence,* ed. A. Tekian, C. H. McGuire, and W. C. McGaghie. Chicago: Department of Medical Education, University of Illinois at Chicago.

McLaughlin, K., and H. Mandin. 2001. A schematic approach to diagnosing and resolving lecturalgia. *Med Educ* 35:1135–42.

McLean, M., F. Cilliers, and J. M. Van Wyk. 2008. AMEE Guide No. 36. Faculty development: Yesterday, today and tomorrow. *Med Teach* 30:555–84.

Mellis, C. M. 2008. Optimizing training: What clinicians have to offer and how to deliver it. *Paediat Resp Rev* 9:105–13.

Michaelsen, L. K., and M. Sweet. 2008a. The essential elements of team-based learning. In *Team-Based Learning: Small Groups' Learning's Next Big Step.* New Directions for Teaching and Learning, ed. L. K. Michaelsen, M. Sweet, and D. X. Parmelee, 7–27. San Francisco: Jossey-Bass.

Michaelsen, L. K., and M. Sweet. 2008b. Fundamental principles and practices of team-based learning. In *Team-Based Learning for Health Professions Education,* ed. L. K. Michaelsen, D. X. Parmelee, K. K. McMahon, and R. E. Levine, 9–34. Sterling, VA: Stylus Publishing.

Miller, G. E. 1990. Assessment of clinical skills/competence/performance. *Acad Med* 65:S63–67.

Mittal, R. D., and D. H. Balaban. 1997. The esophagogastric junction. *N Engl J Med* 336:924–32.

Morrison, E. H. 2002. An Objective Structured Teaching Examination (OSTE) for Generalist Resident Physicians. Available through the Residents' Teaching Skills Web site, a collaboration with the Graduate Medical Education Section of the Association of American Medical Colleges. www.ucimc.netouch.com/contact.htm.

Morrison, E. H., J. R. Boker, J. Hollingshead, M. D. Prislin, M. A. Hitchcock, and D. K. Litzelman. 2002. Reliability and validity of an objective structured teaching examination for generalist resident teachers. *Acad Med* 77:S29–32.

Morse, C. B. 2009. Becoming a team. *Acad Med* 84:781.

Mueller, P. S., S. C. Litin, M. L. Sowden, T. M. Habermann, and N. F. LaRusso. 2003. Strategies for improving attendance at medical grand rounds at an academic medical center. *Mayo Clin Proc* 78:549–53.

Mueller, P. S., C. M. Segovis, S. C. Litin, T. M. Habermann, and T. A. Parrino. 2006. Current status of medical grand rounds in departments of medicine at US medical schools. *Mayo Clin Proc* 81:313–21.

Naftulin, D. H., J. E. Ware, and F. A. Donnelly. 1973. The Doctor Fox Lecture: A paradigm of educational seduction. *J Med Educ* 48:630–35.

National Board of Medical Examiners. Constructing written test questions for the basic and clinical sciences. www.nbme.org/about/itemwriting.asp.

Neher, J. O., K. C. Gordon, B. Meyer, and N. Stevens. 1992. A five-step "microskills" model of clinical teaching. *J Am Board Fam Prac* 5:419–24.

Newble, D., and R. Cannon. 1987. *A Handbook for Medical Teachers.* 2nd ed., 54–67. Lancaster, UK: MTP Press.

Nicholson, L. J., and L. Y. Shieh. 2005. Teaching evidence-based medicine on a busy hospitalist service: Residents rate a pilot curriculum. *Acad Med* 80:607–9.

Norcini, J. J., L. L. Blank, G. J. Arnold, and H. R. Kimball. 1995. The Mini-CEX (Clinical Evaluation Exercise): A preliminary investigation. *Ann Intern Med* 123:795–99.

Norcini, J. J., L. L. Blank, D. Duffy, and G. S. Fortna. 2003. The mini-CEX: A method for assessing clinical skills. *Ann Intern Med* 138:476–81.

Osborn, L. M., and N. Whitman. 1991. *Ward Attending: The Forty-Day Month.* Salt Lake City: Department of Family and Preventive Medicine, University of Utah School of Medicine.

Osler, W. 1901. The natural method of teaching the subject of medicine. *JAMA* 36:1673–79.

Palmer, P. J. 2007. *The Courage to Teach: Exploring the Inner Landscape of a Teacher's Life.* 10th ed. San Francisco: John Wiley & Sons.

Pangaro, L. N., and W. C. McGaghie. 2005. Evaluation and grading of students. In *Guidebook for Clerkship Directors.* 3rd ed., ed. R.-M. E. Fincher, 133–248. Omaha, NE: Alliance for Clinical Education.

Papadakis, M. A., A. Teherani, M. A. Banach, T. R. Knettler, S. L. Rattner, D. T. Stern, J. J. Veloski, and C. S. Hodgson. 2005. Disciplinary action by medical boards and prior behavior in medical school. *N Engl J Med* 353:2673–82.

Papp, K. K., J. N. Aucott, and D. C. Aron. 2001. The problem of retaining clinical teachers in academic medicine. *Perspect Biol Med* 44:402–13.

Parmelee, D. X. 2008. Team-based learning in health professions education: Why is it a good fit? In *Team-Based Learning for Health Professions Education,* ed. L. K. Michaelsen, D. X. Parmelee, K. K. McMahon, and R. E. Levine, 3–8. Sterling, VA: Stylus Publishing.

Parmelee, D. X., D. DeStephen, and N. J. Borges. 2009. Medical students' attitudes about team-based learning in a pre-clinical curriculum. *Med Educ Online* 14:1–7.

Paulman, P. M., J. L. Susman, and C. A. Abboud. 2000. *Precepting Medical Students in the Office.* Baltimore: Johns Hopkins University Press.

Pinsky, L. E., D. Monson, and D. M. Irby. 1998. How excellent teachers are made: Reflecting on success to improve teaching. *Adv Health Sci Educ Theory Pract* 3:207–15.

Pugsley, L. 2009. How to approach writing for publication in medical education. *Educ Prim Care* 20:122–24.

Quinn, C. T., and A. J. Rush. 2009. Writing and publishing your research findings. *J Investig Med* 57:634–39.

Quirk, M. E. 2006. *Intuition and Metacognition in Medical Education: Keys to Developing Expertise.* New York: Springer Publishing Co.

Quirk, M., K. Mazor, H.-L. Haley, S. Wellman, D. Keller, D. Hatem, and L. A. Keller. 2005. Reliability and validity of checklists and global ratings by standardized students, trained raters, and faculty raters in an Objective Structured Teaching Exercise (OSTE). *Teach Learn Med* 17:202–9.

Ramani, S. 2006. Twelve tips to promote excellence in medical teaching. *Med Teach* 28:19–23.

Reed, D. N., Jr., T. A. Littman, C. I. Anderson, G. R. Dirani, J. M. Gauvin, K. N. Apelgren, and C. A. Slomski. 2008. What is an hour-lecture worth? *Am J Surg* 195:379–81.

Regehr, G. 2004. Trends in medical education research. *Acad Med* 79:939–47.

Reichsman, F., F. E. Browning, and J. R. Hinshaw. 1964. Observations of undergraduate clinical teaching in action. *J Med Educ* 39:147–63.

Reynolds, R. J., and C. S. Candler. 2008. MedEdPortal: Educational scholarship for teaching. *J Continu Ed Health Prof* 28:91–94.

Robins, L., D. Ambrozy, and L. E. Pinsky. 2006. Promoting academic excellence through leadership development at the University of Washington: The Teaching Scholars Program. *Acad Med* 81:979–83.

Rubenstein, W., and Y. Talbot. 1992. *Medical Teaching in Ambulatory Care: A Practical Guide.* New York: Springer Publishing Co.

Saha, S., G. Guiton, P. F. Wimmers, and L. Wilkerson. 2008. Student body racial and ethnic composition and diversity-related outcomes in US medical schools. *JAMA* 300:1135–45.

Sands, D. Z., and J. B. McGee. 2001. Presenting your work: Designing presentations, using technology, and giving the show. http://home.caregroup.org/clinical/docs/presenting_your_work.doc.

Satterlee, W. G., R. G. Eggers, and D. A. Grimes. 2008. Effective medical education: Insights from the Cochrane Library. *Obstet Gyn Surv* 63:329–33.

Schuwirth, L. W. T., and C. P. M. van der Vleuten. 2005. Written assessments. In *A Practical Guide for Medical Teachers,* ed. J. A. Dent and R. M. Harden, 311–22. London: Elsevier/Churchill Livingston.

Scott, D. J., E. M. Ritter, S. T. Tesfay, E. A. Pimentel, A. Nagji, and G. M. Fried. 2008. Certification pass rate of 100% for fundamentals of laparoscopic surgery skills after proficiency-based training. *Surg Endosc* 22:1887–93.

Sequist, T. D. 2009. *Addressing Racial Disparities in Health Care: A Targeted Action Plan for Academic Medical Centers*. Washington, DC: Association of American Medical Colleges.

Shea, J. A., L. Arnold, and K. V. Mann. 2004. A RIME perspective on the quality and relevance of current and future medical education research. *Acad Med* 79:931–38.

Shields, H. M., D. Guss, S. C. Somers, B. P. Kerfoot, B. S. Mandell, W. J. Travassos, S. M. Ullman, S. Maroo, J. P. Honan, L. W. Raymond, E. M. Goldberg, D. A. Leffler, J. N. Hayward, S. R. Pelletier, A. R. Carbo, L. N. Fishman, B. J. Nath, M. A. Cohn, and J. P. Hafler. 2007. A faculty development program to train tutors to be discussion leaders rather than facilitators. *Acad Med* 82:486–92.

Shields, H. M., D. A. Leffler, A. A. White III, J. P. Hafler, S. R. Pelletier, R. P. O'Farrell, R. Llerena-Quinn, J. N. Hayward, S. Salamone, A. M. Lenco, P. G. Blanco, and A. S. Peters. 2009. Integration of racial, cultural, ethnic, and socioeconomic factors into a gastrointestinal pathophysiology course. *Clin Gastroenterol Hepatol* 7:279–84.

Shields, H. M., V. E. Nambudiri, D. A. Leffler, C. Akileswaran, E. R. Gurrola, R. Jimenez, A. Saltzman, P. A. Samuel, K. Wong, A. A. White III, J. P. Hafler, J. N. Hayward, S. R. Pelletier, R. P. O'Farrell, P. G. Blanco, S. M. Kappler, and R. Ilerena-Quinn. 2009. Using medical students to assess cross-cultural triggers for case discussion in a preclinical pathophysiology tutorial. *Kaohsiung J Med Sci* 25:493–502.

Shumway, J. M., and R. M. Harden. 2003. AMEE Guide No. 25: The assessment of learning outcomes for the competent and reflective physician. *Med Teach* 25:569–584.

Sidorov, J. 1995. How are internal medicine residency journal clubs organized and what makes them successful? *Arch Intern Med* 155:1193–97.

Simpson, D. E., and R.-M. Fincher. 1999. Making a case for the teaching scholar. *Acad Med* 74:1296–99.

Sisco, B. R. 1998. Forum, panel, and symposium. In *Adult Learning Methods: A Guide for Effective Instruction*. 2nd ed., ed. M. W. Galbraith, 260–64. Malabar, FL: Krieger Publishing Co.

Skeff, K. M. 1988. Enhancing teaching effectiveness and vitality in the ambulatory setting. *J Gen Intern Med* 3 (Suppl.):S26–33.

Skeff, K. M. 2007. The chromosomal analysis of teaching: the search for promoter genes. *Trans Am Clin Climatol Assoc* 118:123–32.

Smith, S. R., and R. Dollase. 1999. AMEE Guide No. 14: Outcome-based education: Part 2—Planning, implementing and evaluating a competency-based curriculum. *Med Teach* 21:15–21.

Spady, W. G. 1994. *Outcome-Based Education: Critical Issues and Answers*. Arlington, VA: American Association of School Administrators.

Steele, D. J., J. D. Medder, and P. Turner. 2000. A comparison of learning outcomes and attitudes in student-versus faculty-led problem-based learning: An experimental study. *Med Educ* 34:23–29.

Steinert, Y., L. Nasmith, P. J. McLeod, and L. Conochie. 2003. A teaching scholars program to develop leaders in medical education. *Acad Med* 78:142–49.

Steinert, Y., K. Mann, A. Centeno, D. Dolmans, J. Spencer, M. Gelula, and D. Prideaux 2006. A systematic review of faculty development initiatives designed to improve teaching effectiveness in medical education: BEME guide No. 8. *Med Teach* 28:497–526.

Steinert, Y., P. J. McLeod, S. Liben, and L. Snell. 2008. Writing for publication in medical education: The benefits of a faculty development workshop and peer writing group. *Med Teach* 30:e280–85.

Steinmann, A. F., N. M. Dy, G. C. Kane, J. I. Kennedy, S. Silbiger, N. Sharma, and W. Rifkin. 2009. APM Perspectives. The modern teaching physician-responsibilities and challenges: An APDIM white paper. *Am J Med* 122:692–97.

Stern, D. T., B. C. Williams, A. Gill, L. D. Gruppen, J. O. Woolliscroft, and C. M. Grum. 2000. Is there a relationship between attending physicians' and residents' teaching skills and students' examination scores? *Acad Med* 75:1144–46.

Stuart, M. R., and P. S. Krauser. 2000. Using goals and objectives in community rotations. In *Precepting Medical Students in the Office,* ed. P. M. Paulman, J. L. Susman, and C. A. Abboud, 62–65. Baltimore: Johns Hopkins University Press.

Sutkin, G., E. Wagner, I. Harris, and R. Schiffer. 2008. What makes a good clinical teacher in medicine? A review of the literature. *Acad Med* 83:452–66.

Taylor, D., and B. Miflin. 2008. Problem-based learning: Where are we now? *Med Teach* 30:742–63.

Tavakol, M., R. Dennick, and S. Tavakol. 2009. A descriptive study of medical educators' views of problem-based learning. BMC *Med Educ* 9:66. www.biomedcentral.com/1472–6920/9/66.

Teunissen, P. W., and T. Dornan. 2008. Lifelong learning at work. *BMJ* 336:667–69.

Thibault, G. E., J. M. Neill, and D. H. Lowenstein. 2003. The Academy at Harvard Medical School: Nurturing, teaching and stimulating innovation. *Acad Med* 78:673–81.

Thomas, P. A. 2009. Goals and objectives. In *Curriculum Development for Medical Education.* 2nd ed., ed. D. E. Kern, P. A. Thomas, and M. T. Hughes, 43–56. Baltimore: Johns Hopkins University Press.

Thomas, P. A., M. Diener-West, M. I. Canto, D. R. Martin, W. S. Post, and M. B. Streiff. 2004. Results of an academic promotion and career path survey of faculty at the Johns Hopkins University School of Medicine. *Acad Med* 79:258–64.

Tiberius, R. G. 1990. *Small Group Teaching: A Trouble-shooting Guide.* Monograph Series 22. Toronto: Ontario Institute for Studies in Education.

Tosteson, D. C., S. J. Adelstein, and S. T. Carver, eds. 1994. *New Pathways to Medical Education: Learning to Learn at Harvard Medical School.* Cambridge, MA: Harvard University Press.

Turner, J. L., and M. E. Dankoski. 2008. Objective structured clinical exams: A critical review. *Fam Med* 40:574–78.

Viggiano, T. R., C. Shub, and R. W. Giere. 2000. The Mayo Clinic's Clinician-Educator Award: A program to encourage educational innovation and scholarship. *Acad Med* 75:940–43.

Wachter, R. M. and L. Goldman. 2002. The Hospitalist movement 5 years later. *JAMA* 287:487–94.

Wachter, R. M., P. Katz, J. Showstack, A. B. Bindman, and L. Goldman. 1998. Reorganizing an academic medical service: Impact on cost, quality, patient satisfaction, and education. *JAMA* 279:1560–65.

Wamsley, M., K. Julian, E. Morrison, and S. Zabar. 2006. Workshop F06: Introduction to the Objective Structured Teaching Evaluation (OSTE): A Novel Tool for Evaluating

Teaching Skills. Los Angeles: Society of General Internal Medicine. www.sgim.org/userfiles/file/AMHandouts/AM06/handouts/WF06.pdf.

Wayne, D. B., J. Butter, V. J. Siddall, M. J. Fudala, L. A. Lindquist, J. Feinglass, L. D. Wade, and W. C. McGahie. 2005. Simulation-based training of internal medicine residents in advanced cardiac life support protocols: A randomized trial. *Teach Learn Med* 17:210–16.

Weinberger, S. E., L. G. Smith, and V. U. Collier, Education Committee of the American College of Physicians. 2006. Redesigning training for internal medicine. *Ann Intern Med* 144:927–32.

Weinholtz, D., and J. C. Edwards. 1992. *Teaching during Rounds: A Handbook for Attending Physicians and Residents*. Baltimore: Johns Hopkins University Press.

West, J. B. 2002. Thoughts on teaching physiology to medical students in 2002. *Physiologist* 45:389–93.

Westberg, J., and H. Jason. 1991. *Making Effective Presentations*. User's Guide. A CIS Video Program for Teachers in the Health Professions. Boulder, CO: Center for Instructional Support.

Westberg, J., and H. Jason. 2001. *Fostering Reflection and Providing Feedback: Helping Others Learn from Experience*. New York: Springer Publishing Co.

Wetzel, M. S. 1994. Problem-based learning: An update on problem-based learning at Harvard Medical School. *Ann Comm-Oriented Educ* 7:237–47.

Wetzel, M. S., and L. M. Reid. 1991. The Multistation Exercise: Accessible, Adaptable, Active Learning. Association of American Medical Colleges annual meeting, Washington, DC.

Wetzel, M. S., T. J. Kaptchuk, and D. M. Eisenberg. 2003. Complementary and alternative medical therapies: Implications for medical education. *Ann Intern Med* 138:191–96.

Whalley, S. 2000. *How to Write Powerful Letters of Recommendation*. Minneapolis: Educational Media Corp.

Whelan, J. S. 2009. *Introduction to Evidence-based Medicine*. Video tutorial providing background on the rationale for evidence-based medicine (EBM) and the process of EBM practice. http://hms.harvard.libguides.com/ebm.

Whitaker, T. 2004. *What Great Teachers Do Differently: Fourteen Things That Matter Most*. Larchmont, NY: Eye on Education.

Whitman, N. 1990. *Creative Medical Teaching*. Salt Lake City: Department of Family and Preventive Medicine, University of Utah School of Medicine.

Whitman, N., and T. L. Schwenk. 1997. *The Physician as Teacher*. 2nd ed. Salt Lake City: Whitman Associates.

Wilkerson, L., and D. M. Irby. 1998. Strategies for improving teaching practices: A comprehensive approach to faculty development. *Acad Med* 73:387–96.

Williamson, J. C., S. L. Schrop, and A. J. Costa. 2008. Awarding faculty rank to non-tenured physician faculty in a consortium medical school. *Fam Med* 40:32–39.

Winston, P. 2007a. *How to Speak: Lecture Tips from Patrick Winston*. Disc 5. Derek Bok Center Series on College Teaching. Cambridge, MA: Derek Bok Center for Teaching and Learning, Harvard University.

Winston, P. 2007b. *Technically Speaking: Making Complex Matters Simple*. Disc 5. Derek Bok Center Series on College Teaching. Cambridge, MA: Derek Bok Center for Teaching and Learning, Harvard University.

Wood, D. F. 2003. Problem-based learning. *BMJ* 326:328–30.

Wood, W. B. 2004. Clickers: A teaching gimmick that works. *Dev Cell* 7:796–98.

Wright, S. M., D. E. Kern, K. Kolodner, D. M. Howard, and F. L. Brancati. 1998. Attributes of excellent attending-physician role models. *N Engl J Med* 339:1986–93.

Young, L., A. Orlandi, B. Galichet, and H. Heussler. 2009. Effective teaching and learning on the wards: Easier said than done? *Med Educ* 43:808–17.

Zerzan, J. T., R. Hess, E. Schur, R. S. Phillips, and N. Rigotti. 2009. Making the most of mentors: A guide for mentees. *Acad Med* 84:140–44.

Zimmerman, R. K., F. L. Ruben, and E. R. Ahwesh. 2005. *Teaching Immunization for Medical Education*. Washington, DC: Association of Teachers of Preventive Medicine.

Index

case histories. *See* clinical cases
chair's letter of recommendation, 252–53
chief residencies, 21
Chopra, Sanjiv, 204
Christensen, Clay M., 207
Cleveland Clinic Lerner College of Medicine, 74
clickers. *See* audience-response systems
clinical cases: case-based small-group learning and, 167; cross-cultural care and, 187–88; example of, 108–9; grand rounds and, 166; inpatient teaching and, 137, 145; in mini-cases and focused discussions, 123–28, 124*fig*; problem-based learning and, 105–6, 112–13; time constraints and, 223; writing of, 106–8
Clinical Evaluation Exercises (CEXs), 148
Clinical Gastroenterology and Hepatology, 27, 227
Clinical-level teaching: feedback and, 65, 84–87; integrated multistation exercises and, 190–92; learning objectives and, 55–56; out-patient teaching and, 151–55; recognition for, 212–13. *See also* inpatient teaching
clinical practice, 208–9
clinical skills, 8–9, 139–40
Clinical Skills examination (CS), 77
Clinical Teacher, 27
collaboration, 198, 209–10, 229–30
Collier, V. U., 151
Collins, J., 66–67
Committee of Human Studies (Harvard Medical School), 232
communication skills, 76–77, 140, 141, 186, 200
comprehension (Bloom's taxonomy), 54–55, 66, 69–70
"A Concept of Critical Thinking" (Ennis), 56
consent forms, 226, 231–32, 233–34, 234*t*
courses in medical education, 22–25
Critical Appraisal Tool software, 194–95
critical thinking, 52, 56–58
cross-cultural care, 186–89, 203
Crumlish, C. M., 140
cueing (in questions), 68
culturally competent care, 186–89
curricula vitae (CVs), 245–46, 249–50
curriculum development, 52–54, 58–62, 74, 248
curriculum implementation, 61

Dankoski, M. E., 76
Dannefer, E. F., 74
DAVE project, 23
Davis, M. H., 214
Deenadayalan, Y., 193
Dent, J. A., 151
disabilities, 73
Dorfsman, M. L., 149

educational research projects: authorship and, 229–30; career advancement and, 9–10, 24–25; data collection and analysis for, 230–31, 234–35; funding, 231; Institutional Review Board and, 231–34, 243*t*; meeting abstracts and, 239–41; overview of, 226–29; publication of, 235–39, 241–42
educational terms, 52
education symposia, 25
Ende, J., 80, 86–87
Ennis, R. H., 56–58
essay questions, 70–71
Essential Evidence-Based Medicine, 135
evaluation (Bloom's Taxonomy), 54–55, 66, 68, 140
evaluations by students, 45–46, 61–62, 66, 95, 172. *See also* feedback
evaluations of students, 83–84, 87. *See also* feedback to students
evidence-based medicine, 135–36
Evidence-Based Medicine Working Group, 135
examination question types, 65–71
exams. *See* learner assessment
expectations, 64, 84, 137–39, 155, 157, 229
experience, 138, 144–45
exploration, 38, 99*t*, 99–100, 103, 114
exposition, 99*t*, 99, 103, 114

faculty development: cross-cultural care and, 188–89; fellowships/courses in medical education, 22–25; objective structured teaching exercises and, 195–96; tutor development and, 109–12
failing exams, 71–73
favoritism, 15
Federman, Daniel, 118
feedback: curriculum development and, 61–62; objective structured teaching exercises and,

About the Author

Helen M. Shields received her bachelor of arts degree in biological sciences from Mount Holyoke College, in South Hadley, Massachusetts, and her medical degree from Tufts University Medical School, in Boston. She did her internship and first-year residency in medicine at Tufts–New England Medical Center, in Boston, and was a senior resident and subsequently chief resident in medicine at New York Hospital–Cornell Medical Center, in New York City. Dr. Shields did her fellowship in gastroenterology at the University of Pennsylvania, in Philadelphia.

Dr. Shields was on the faculty in the division of gastroenterology at Washington University and Barnes Hospital, in St. Louis, as an instructor and then assistant professor of medicine, before coming to Harvard Medical School and Beth Israel Deaconess Medical Center, where she is an associate professor of medicine. She began her academic career as a clinician-researcher but changed to the teacher-clinician track in 1994, when she was asked to be director of the gastrointestinal pathophysiology course for second-year medical students, a position she still holds. In 2001, Dr. Shields was appointed associate master of the Oliver Wendell Holmes Society, an advising and mentoring position in one of the five Harvard Medical School societies.

Dr. Shields won the Harvard Faculty Prize for Excellence in Teaching, awarded by the Faculty Council at Harvard Medical School, in 1999 and again in 2008. In 2003, she won the S. Robert Stone Award for Excellence in Teaching and Clinical Service from the Beth Israel Deaconess Medical Center and Harvard Medical School. She was awarded the Best Preclinical Instructor Award by the Harvard Medical School graduating classes of 2004 and 2007. Dr. Shields received the Excellence in Tutoring Award from the Academy for Teaching and Learning at Harvard Medical School in 2007, 2008, and 2009. She received the Mentor Recognition Award for Medical Student Mentoring from the American Medical Association's–Women's Physicians Congress in 2007 and 2009. In 2010 she was elected education and training councillor of the governing board of the American Gastroenterological Association for 2010 to 2013.